BARREN

a shared journey of infertility, loss, and faith

HEATHER LAVIGNE

Heather's book, *Barren: A Shared Journey of Infertility, Loss, and Faith*, is a powerful testament to the strength of the human spirit and the steadfast love of God. Through her vulnerability, courage, and unshakable faith, she gives voice to countless women and families walking the path of infertility — a journey marked by both heartbreak and hope.

Her story beautifully reminds us that science and faith are not opposing forces, but partners in healing. It is an honor to know that CNY Fertility played a small role in her family's story, and I am humbled by her trust in us during such sacred moments.

Heather's words will comfort those who feel alone, restore hope to those still waiting, and point every heart toward the infinite love that brings new life in all its forms.

\- Robert Kiltz, MD

Founder & CEO, CNY Fertility

Infertility and loss can make you feel like you're carrying something no one else can see. As I read Heather's story, even though our journeys are different, I saw pieces of my own experience in her words. She's honest about the hard parts and points you back to God in a way that feels steady and true.

If you're walking through infertility, miscarriage, or a long season of waiting, this book will meet you right where you are. Heather reminds you that you're seen, you're loved, and you're not forgotten. I'm grateful she wrote this.

\- Nicole Clark

Founder, Twelve 12 Ministries

Barren is a needed tender companion for anyone navigating the silent ache of infertility and loss. Rooted in biblical truth, it reminds us that even in the waiting, God is near.

\- Rev. Beth Caulfield

Pastor, author and director of
the movie *Conceivable*.

BARREN

HEATHER LAVIGNE

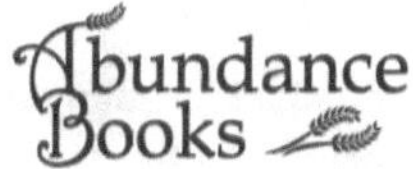

ISBN: 978-1-963377-9-0

Library of Congress Control Number: 2026904264

Abundance Books
Kalamazoo, Michigan
www.abundance-books.com

Printed in the United States of America

10 9 8 7 6 5 4 3 2 1

Cover design by Amber Weigand-Buckley, Barefaced Media
Interior design and layout by Taryn Golliher

Dedicated to my three little Ebenezers: Dax, Bodie, and Violet, who are a constant reminder of God's faithfulness. To my four loves in Jesus's arms, He is the only one who loves you more than I do. And to Brent-my journey begins and ends with you. I love you so much.

May the words of my mouth and the meditation
of my heart be pleasing in your sight,
O Lord, my Rock and my Redeemer.
Psalm 19:14

Acknowledgements

I never would have thought it possible in the days I typed out my story in stream of consciousness that it would come to this holy ground. It is indeed comparable to birthing a baby. Thank you to Jenn DaFoe-Turner, Teresa Janzen, and Abundance Books for believing in this "project". I'll never forget the day I sat knee to knee with you at SpeakUp. When I finished sharing my story, you looked straight into my tear-filled eyes and said, "This must be published."

Thank you to SpeakUp for the tools, teaching, encouragement, and sacred worship that ushered me into His presence and calling.

Heartfelt thanks to my pool I kept small who were willing to climb in the dark waters with me- Kate Veenstra, Lynsey Leep, Amy Ludwigson, Erin O'Donohue, Angie Stumpo, Barb Baumann, Maureen Abid, Lisa Granger, Lisa Lago, Ashley Verhey, Sarah DePas, Karen Lindhout, and Heide Rollings. What a great gift you were and continue to be in my life.

I would have never gotten to a place of restoration without church support. To my small group from Magnify and Magnify church family as well as my Beloved and TLC Church family who have provided tremendous support and healing along the way.

To Dr. LG for taking gentle care of my body and heart. To Dr. Kiltz and CNY Fertility for their tenacity and heart for their patients.

Finally, to the woman reading this who feels shamed or cursed by her circumstances: this book is for you. Barrenness in body or heart is never the end of the story. God deeply loves you and is with you.

With deep gratitude,
Heather

Contents

Before We Begin

Jour · ney /'jərnē/ n.

1. An act of traveling from one place to another.
2. A distance, course, or area traveled.
3. Passage or progress from one stage to another.

I would guess the reason you picked up this book is because you are on a journey. It's a journey you didn't ask for. To a place you never dreamed you would have to travel to. The distance feels never-ending, peaked with high hopes and soul-sucking plummets. It's a passage marked with endless forms to fill out, invasions of privacy, flawed (but often well-intentioned) advice, and self-protective retreats. The trip might have started out with a van load full of support, but now it feels a little lonely. You have been banged up a bit, but have weathered out the storm so far. Still, you can't shake the sense that your faith feels like it's sinking, and hope feels too slippery to hold. Maybe you have gotten to a point where you feel like you can't go on.

Perhaps you are the husband, sister, family member, or friend just reaching for straws of understanding to try to relate to your person. Bless you for deeply loving your dear one in this season; your presence is critical. I am so glad you are here.

I've been on this road you are on. I know the unexpected bumps and frustrating detours well. I've felt the hopeless exhaustion you feel. I've sat next to you at the hospital, the reproductive endocrinologist's clinic, the adoption lawyer's office, the therapist's practice, your pastor's study, and the waiting room we all feel eternally trapped in… the one where we wait for our baby. And so, I wrote this book for women, their families, and loved ones because I know the stigma, love, pain, and joy that comes on this hopeful road to parenthood. And I believe deeply that this road is a little easier when walked alongside someone else.

I know I called it a journey, but when I look back at how it felt to walk those roads, I did not feel like I was progressing or even moving forward. Most times, I felt like I was stuck or even drifting backward. Backward in my relationships, my friendships, my marriage, my mental health, my physical well-being, and in my trust in God. I deeply wrestled with why God had allowed this incredible hardship into my life. As the years passed and my health unraveled before me, so did my confidence in God's goodness and sovereignty. Why did He allow this journey to go on and on? Why did it have to be so very visible? Why wasn't anything working? Why was my body failing to do what He so beautifully created it to do?

I built a fortress around my heart. I dug in deeply, trying to understand the Lord's will while fighting with my own. I tried to read the Bible, but often stumbled upon what I felt were less than encouraging words:

- "Be fruitful and increase in number" (Genesis 1:28 NIV).
- "He will bless the fruit of your womb" (Deuteronomy 7:13 NIV).
- "Children are a heritage from the LORD, the fruit of the womb a reward…. Blessed is the man who fills his quiver with them!" (Psalm 127:3, 5 ESV).
- "I will look on you with favor and make you fruitful and increase your numbers, and I will keep my covenant with you" (Leviticus 26:9 NIV).

To be honest, every time I read or heard those verses, my heart became a little more hardened. They were contrary to my own circumstances—I couldn't help but wonder if God, the universe, and my own body were actively withholding something from me. My heart had begun to believe the lies that the enemy whispered in my ear… *Did God really say He wants good things for you? How could this be His will? Surely you have done something wrong, this must be punishment.*

If you're on this journey, I want you to know this: It is not your fault. You are not cursed or forgotten, and you are not alone. Even though it may feel that way sometimes.

To understand why this pain exists, we have to go back to a place and a time where brokenness first entered the human story. It traces all the way back to the Garden of Eden when Adam and Eve ate from the Tree of the Knowledge of Good and Evil. The serpent caused Eve to doubt what God had instructed, to question if God was withholding knowledge from her; she ate the fruit, as did Adam. Sin entered a perfect world. The consequence of that sin still affects our world today—separation from God, the curse upon the ground, and pain in childbirth. But let's explore the last one a bit more.

"To the woman he said, 'I will make your pains in childbearing very severe; with painful labor you will give birth to children'" (Genesis 3:16 NIV).

I've always understood the curse of birthing pains to be literal. However, the understanding of this pain changes depending on Bible translation. The King James version reads, "I will greatly multiply thy sorrow and thy conception, in sorrow thou shalt bring forth children." The Amplified version (AMPC) captures it this way: "I will greatly multiply your grief and your suffering in pregnancy and the pangs of childbearing." You might wonder, as I did, why are we talking about sorrow and grief at the time of childbirth? Shouldn't that have been a joyful time? To sort this all out, scholars go back to the original Hebrew. Stay with me. It's going to get a little Old Testament geeky, but it will be worth it in the end. The phrase "pains in childbearing" originates from the Hebrew word *itsabon*. While there are many Hebrew words for labor pains, *itsabon* is not one of them. *Itsabon* best translates to toil or difficult struggle. This is evident in verse 18 where *itsabon* depicts the frustration and hardship Adam would experience working the land. The root word of *itsabon* is *'otseb* or *'etseb*, and these words appear often in the Bible (2 Samuel 19:1-2 NIV, Proverbs 15:1 NASB, Proverbs 10:22 NIV, Psalm 147:2-3 NIV). The meaning behind them is understood as feelings of emotional grief and hurtfulness. The oldest translation of the Bible is telling us childbirth was to be associated with the grief of toil and hurtful struggle. Why? Let's go a bit further.

Herayon, the Hebrew word translated as childbirth, is more commonly used for the process up to conception and all events following. It's all making sense now. The curse of Eve encompasses the entire journey toward motherhood: "the agony, hardship, worry, and anxiety of the circumstances in which children are conceived, born and raised, and in which they die…" (Mackie, 2024).

It is not just the physical pain of birthing a child. It's the grief of not being able to conceive; it's not being chosen by a biologic parent, it's the negative tests after a monitored cycle, the cancelled IVF (in vitro fertilization) cycles, the hopeless chemical pregnancies, the soul stealing second trimester miscarriages, the unspeakable pain of a stillbirth, and the devastating death of a premature baby. So, when we ask, *Why? Why is this happening to me?* We must consider this world was cursed from the beginning of time. That curse did not start with you or me. It was never just our burden to bear. The groans of creation echo from every family who bears the weight of grief, long-suffering, and disappointment relating to loss and infertility. There is a deep longing for the restoration of life and hope that only God can bring.

While it's often difficult to read scripture that celebrates childbearing, the Bible ultimately tells a greater narrative of God's great love for His people. The pages of the Old and New Testaments are lined with stories of enduring grief born from infertility and loss. God saw it fit to tell *His* story through the lives of His beloved women just as I believe He sees it fit to tell His story through us. The lineage of His chosen people and His promise began in infertility. Abraham and Sarah, Isaac and Rebekah, Jacob and Rachel…were all families that suffered from barren seasons. He chose to grow their hearts for Him before He grew their families.

We will study the lives of these women and find they felt forgotten, cursed, and disgraced. They were commonly referred to as "barren." During biblical times, there was immense pressure to produce a family even greater than what we experience today. Being childless outright contradicted God's instruction. Remember He commanded Noah to be fruitful, to fill the earth, and subdue it. Fruitfulness was linked to a family's legacy and livelihood. No children meant no caretakers for aging parents and no heirs.

In that time, barren women were viewed with suspicion— believed to be possibly diseased or infidels. Being frequently cast out, these women were at risk of slavery and poverty. Even amid so much adversity, many remained resilient in faith, offering us strength and solidarity for our own journeys.

Many dealt with impatience, family turmoil, bitterness, and envy. They struggled to be faithful to God while enduring shame from their family members and community. They were women who tried to push through and act like they were fine, they were overlooked, they were women who wrestled with God's goodness and seeming lack of mercy. Maybe this sounds like you because I know it sounded like me. These stories will serve as a roadmap to find the God of comfort, the God of provision, and the God of goodness when we struggle to find meaning in the dark.

My Story

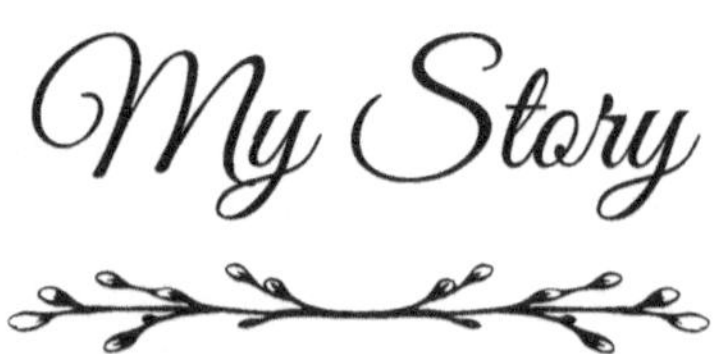

As we study these women, I will weave in snapshots and deeper reflections from my own experiences with infertility and loss, but the broader strokes I will share with you here. I want to give a gentle trigger warning. The following section is my personal account of infertility and the loss of our four babies, which may be sensitive for some readers to take in. Tend to your heart while you read—pause, skip ahead, or return as needed.

So here goes, from the beginning. In the fall of 2010, I married the love of my life, Brent, under trees bursting with autumn leaves. Our wedding pictures show our young faces flushed from the October chill. We were bright-eyed with exhilaration of the unknown road ahead. We started out like many do: career-driven, not really thinking about when or how we would grow our family. There would be plenty of time for that later. But about two years after the goalie was pulled, we started to scratch our heads over why the inevitable wasn't happening. I visited a local recommended obstetrician who provided me with a plan for further workup, but said, reassuringly, "You probably won't need that!"

I wished she were right. But six months later, there I was on Clomid (a drug to stimulate ovulation), and it wasn't working. She placed a referral to our local fertility experts and we faltered to schedule the appointment. "Maybe we need just another month," my husband suggested. *Do we need to go through all of that? I don't want IVF,* I thought to myself. Months had already turned to years, though, and small worries grew to a relentless ache for a child. There were the silent, tear-filled car rides home from friends' parties where they announced, "Weeee'reeeee pregnant!" and the stack of baby shower invitations that got pushed to the back of the mail basket. There was the friendship I struggled to be supportive in because I could only see my own empty arms. I knew we needed more intervention, and maybe some solidarity.

So, in addition to the fertility appointments, we started attending local RESOLVE support group meetings. "RESOLVE is a not-for-profit company dedicated to supporting groups challenged by their family-building journey to reach resolution through knowledge, support, and unity" (Resolve, 2025). The group of us laughed and scoffed in disbelief over the ridiculous things people say. We formed a bond around the grief we held close to our hearts. We shared our experiences at the fertility office, where the specialist drew algorithms in tiny chicken scratches showing how long it should take to get pregnant and the treatments it would require. We had all endured the fifteen-minute visit, where we were whisked out the door with a number of lab slips and one large bill.

My husband came to all of these appointments and meetings with me. He was more laid-back about all this. More patient, too. He let me make most of the decisions as my career as a nurse practitioner had lent additional knowledge and background. However, in this case, I surely did not know what was happening to my body. Underneath my steel surface rose an uncertainty that something was really wrong and we were all missing it. So, we did the blood work, we checked the assessment boxes, and we paid the big bills—only to find out there was "nothing wrong." Which led to the next phase of monitored cycles, ultrasounds, and lots and lots of medication.

We went from "there's nothing wrong" to "nothing is working."

As more weeks passed, my heart sank and my body grew weary under the side effects of the medication: fatigue, nausea, weight gain, and irregular menstrual periods. My social life took a hit because my calendar was full of appointments, timed encounters, and insurance calls. My emotional and spiritual well-being cracked under the weight of anxiety, cyclical grief, and lack of results. Disoriented about whether this was really God's plan for us, we decided to take a break from it all.

We stopped everything to refocus on us and contemplate if there was a different way to build our family, even though our hearts quietly wished for a biological baby. We started by attending a local adoption seminar, and we quickly found out the road to adoption was anything but short. The counselors told us to anticipate at least two years before we would possibly get the chance to adopt a baby. And then came the hammer.

"We'd like to have a settled plan on how you plan to become parents before you sign our contract," said the counselor, looking me straight in the eyes. We would have to give up fertility treatments. This was a commitment we could not make with certainty.

Through a referral from our RESOLVE support group, we found another adoption lawyer who was sympathetic to our story and willing to support us pursuing fertility treatments and adoption at the same time. We filled out another pile of forms, endured high-level scrutiny, and wrote a big check (because that's what you did if you wanted to get anywhere in the infertility world). But the eve before the contract was to be dropped off at the lawyer's office, I woke in the middle of the night with horrendous abdominal cramps. I had rolled out of bed and was stumbling to the bathroom when I blacked out in my closet. Something was very wrong. This wasn't the first time I had struggled with menstrual pain. It wasn't, in fact, uncommon for me. I had grown accustomed to it, and it was a natural occurrence for women in my family. But the light bulb went on in my head that we could be dealing with a diagnosis bigger than infertility, and this was likely the root cause of it.

A consult was quickly made with a new gynecologist, Dr. LG. He told me what was happening: Endometriosis, a disease where tissue that lines the uterus abnormally grows outside the uterus. This leads to inflammation and scar tissue formation, which can cause debilitating pain, and other complications including infertility. Dr. LG recommended an urgent one-hour surgery to explore and remove any possible inflammation. Two days later, I awoke from the procedure, panic-stricken, pointing at the clock and asking the nurses why a surgery that was supposed to be one hour had lasted four.

"The doctor will tell you when he sees you." My stomach dropped. I felt a sense of dread, and I prayed to God. *I take it all back,* I told Him. *I'll deal with the infertility somehow, please don't let my body have something seriously wrong.*

They rolled me into the recovery room, where Brent told me it was confirmed I had endometriosis, the most serious form: stage IV. Dr. LG had removed it as best as he could, but everything inside was stuck together with scarring, and only one fallopian tube was open. Dr. LG called later that night to go over his findings. He ended our conversation with a bomb.

"You need to get pregnant," he told me. "Do what you need to do, but you should consider IVF. It's your best chance now, and it will probably help your endometriosis."

I couldn't believe it. How painfully ironic. The very thing my body couldn't do over the past four years was now being recommended as treatment for my new disease. This felt like the depths of despair. I felt numb as our lives seemed to swirl out of control. We had wanted to avoid IVF, and now IVF seemed to be our only chance.

So, back we went to the office of shots and disappointment, and we signed on the line for IVF. We were already financially and emotionally spent, but we were out of options. About two months later, I endured an egg retrieval, which was by far one of the most painful things my body has been through. I gripped my husband's hand so tightly that he thought I would break it as the doctor carefully removed each egg from my body. (I hear they mercifully sedate patients for this procedure these days.)

Deep inside, I held on to a sliver of hope that maybe, just maybe, all of this high-level intervention would actually work. Three of my collected eggs were inseminated, producing two perfect little embryos, which were transferred to my womb within a few days. The doctors told me I could resume normal activities while we waited, including travel. So we went on our previously planned work conference across the country, but before we left, we decided to do a quick at-home pregnancy test to see if our procedure worked. (Yes, they tell you not to do this, but we didn't listen.) Our hearts broke when a negative sign floated in front of us, but a support group friend reassured me it was too soon for this type of test to accurately identify a pregnancy level. We went on our trip and took a battlefield of emotions with us, trying our best to enjoy our time away. Miracle of all miracles, a few days later, I got the call from the fertility nurse letting me know my hormone levels indicated I was pregnant. Our spirits soared. It felt like we could finally breathe; the heartache and effort were worth it. It was hard to believe it was all real. After four years of waiting, I was able to tell my husband he was going to be a dad.

Weeks later, we found out by ultrasound that God gave us a double portion of twins. We had indeed transferred two embryos, but most do not understand that two embryos don't equal two babies. This is a common misconception because, sadly, more often than not, neither embryo thrives. We were shocked to see two gestational sacs on the ultrasound screen at our first viewing. We looked at each other in disbelief. (Brent looked a little pale.) Finally, our prayers had been answered. I was so excited, but I was afraid to be too excited. After all, nothing was guaranteed.

Quickly, my life was overrun with follow-up appointments, blood work, and ultrasounds. Dr. LG sat in front of me once again, now taking over the role of obstetrician and warning us that this would be a high-risk pregnancy. The ultrasounds showed two baby boys growing inside along with placenta previa, a condition where the placenta implants too low in the uterus, partially or completely covering the cervix. This pregnancy must be carefully monitored. I was worried and overwhelmed but reassured that my doctor was confident things were progressing. We were willing to do whatever it took to see these babies to the other side. There would be no exercise, no fermented foods, no MSG, no stress, and minimal travel. We accepted all the limitations without hesitation, despite having no clue what the future held.

At twenty weeks, we told our family during our gender reveal party that I had not just one but two baby boy miracles growing inside of me. We filled a box with blue balloons and painted the words "Baby LaVigne" on the outside. When blue balloons were released in the air, everyone clapped for a boy baby. Seconds later, Brent came downstairs carrying another box that said "Baby LaVigne #2." We recorded their looks of shock and unbridled joy. As the next set of blue balloons floated into the air, it felt wonderfully normal to share the surprise after several months that felt so clinical.

Not long after that, I started experiencing contractions due to an "irritable uterus," and bed rest was added to the plan. The days of low to no activity grew long with uncertainty and anxiety. I still found it hard to believe that I was pregnant, even though my body was rapidly changing every day. I was often surprised by reflections in windows and mirrors that accurately showed my growing belly. I struggled to take milestone pregnancy pictures and engage in baby development apps due to fear of the worst happening. Though things were stable, I still struggled to be confident that this dream could actually come true.

When I could get out of the house, I spent time with grandparents, prepared for the babies, and got more involved in the church we had just joined. Brent and I had become members with the intentions to have faith at the center of our family. We sat before a board of elders, and our papers were stamped. We felt the hand of God in our decisions and waited on Him to provide for us moment by moment through this pregnancy, especially when it felt surreal. When we passed the risky phases of pregnancy into the third trimester, we breathed a sigh of relief. My belly expanded to the size of a beach ball and the discomfort really started to set in. I spent most nights outside in our hot tub set at a low temperature, as it was where I was most comfortable. A C-section was scheduled at thirty-eight weeks of gestation, but the boys decided that date was too late for them. At thirty-seven weeks and three days, I awoke in the early morning hours on a Saturday to find my water had broken. We rushed to the hospital, where I was quickly moved into the operating room.

Within minutes, Dax and Bodie were in my arms. Finally,

my heart could be sure nothing could take them away. It all went so fast that Brent almost didn't make the delivery, but the four of us were all there together at last, safe and sound. My heart was so full! All the scares—the early labor, the discomfort, the insecurities—came to fruition in my arms. I could be confident that our family indeed had grown. The next few months were a blur of sleepless nights, poopy diapers, happy milestone pictures, and transitions. We were overjoyed, marveling at our new life while balancing the work that comes with two babies. The sleepless nights, constant feeds, and endless laundry kept my mind in survival mode. We learned to adapt in a multitude of ways, trying our best to parent two little humans at once. We worked as a sleep-deprived team, waiting for the next sleep regression or curveball when the whole routine would change all over again.

At times, I wrestled with feelings that I was not allowed to experience frustration, depression, or any other condition common to post-partum mothers because I had wanted all of this so badly. I think many of us may be pressed toward shame in these moments. I was grateful for experienced mothers and level-headed friends who helped me to acknowledge that tension and normalize these feelings. But most of all, I was blessed by the unbridled joy that came over me, even in the difficult moments or the middle of the night feedings. I know this is not a natural experience for most, but I believe God had gently changed my perspective because of our journey.

And for a while, I thought my story would end there. It's a nice little story, isn't it? We thought so too. But God had other plans. In less than a year, much to our bewilderment, a pregnancy stick showed two lines when no planning or interventions were done. We felt a new level of overwhelming shock and excitement. I didn't think it was possible! Brent and I could barely process the news. But we squared our shoulders, ready to take on the world of car seats lined three in a row, a warehouse of diapers, and daycare costs threefold.

We told our doctor the good news, and Dr. LG was just as shocked and excited as we were. But our joy didn't last. Soon, we sat in his office facing an ultrasound screen that showed a black hole in my womb. No baby—just an empty space. A "blighted ovum," they called it, which is when a fertilized egg implants in a uterus, but an embryo fails to develop.

I figured a "normal" pregnancy would never be in the cards for me. And not only was it not a normal pregnancy, it was also not a normal miscarriage. Full recovery did not come without the help of medication and a surgical procedure three months later. I was angry, and I felt foolish for letting myself believe that my body could do something it had clearly shown it wasn't capable of. I was left with a lingering, stinging bewilderment as I assumed my years with infertility had ended, but now I felt like I had just been dragged right back. I couldn't understand why God did this. I honestly hadn't even considered the idea of another baby up until this point because our minds and hands were so busy taking care of the boys. But when I lost that baby, I felt a yearning for a third baby that I didn't know was inside of me. And I was heartbroken. Suddenly, something I didn't even know I wanted had been ripped from me, and it left a huge hole in its place, just like my womb.

Over the next five years, I couldn't let go of that dream of a third child. Dr. LG said it seemed like my body could do this on its own now, except it clearly couldn't. After sixteen months of trying, we decided on another round of IVF. We opted to do surgery to remove any residual endometriosis beforehand, since I had already started to have symptoms again. We tried to replicate everything we did in our first pregnancy to promote success, only to have a chemical pregnancy (a very early miscarriage, which is only detectable with a hormone blood test). My reproductive endocrinologists became concerned that there could be other complications affecting my ability to get pregnant, including autoimmune disease. So I underwent another medical workup that was mercifully normal. And once again, we contemplated if this was the end of the road for us. The cost of this journey had become too great on our hearts and wallets, and it was time to stop before it cost us more. We tried our best to move on with life, to accept this was God's plan for us. But in all honesty, none of it felt fair.

Seven months later, we became pregnant again, naturally and

unexpectedly. New feelings of dread and guilt washed over me. There was no room for hope anymore. I was convinced my body could not successfully carry a natural pregnancy without the help of science. I blamed myself for not being more careful because I doubted this pregnancy would end any differently than the last two. Everyone was on high alert. Dr. LG ordered frequent blood tests and ultrasounds. I started on progesterone. Our hopes grew cautiously as we heard a heartbeat and saw a live baby on ultrasound. No blank space—a tiny miracle. But the miracle didn't last. At thirteen weeks, we found out that the baby would not make it into this world. All I had left in me was deep anguish and an undercurrent of anger at the seeming injustice of it all. This late miscarriage was rock bottom for us.

Once again, I had to wrestle with the loss of a pregnancy I didn't even ask for. I could not fathom why God would allow this, given what we had already been through. I was ready to walk away from the faith I so surely thought I knew and the God who claimed He loved me.

But it was God who never gave up on me in His loving kindness, His goodness, His sovereignty. He pursued me when I could hardly look at Him, never mind myself. Somehow days turned to months, and months to years. In that course of time, I sought counseling, holistic therapy geared at healing the mind and body, and I found women just like me who were struggling, who I could walk alongside.

It was one of those trusted women who suggested a referral to a new fertility doctor, over 600 miles away at a clinic called CNY Fertility in New York. It was that recommendation that would be the final bend in the winding road of our story. Dr. Kiltz, known as a bleeding heart for infertile families, offered state-of-the-art fertility care, nearly at cost. My friend recommended his funny YouTube videos which provided extensive free education, and his unhurried, peaceful presence. We spent months contemplating whether we had it in us to go back to fertility treatments. We tried out Dr. Kiltz's recommended supplements and diet. We were led to a quiet reassurance that God was leading us to close this chapter with CNY's help. We had nine remaining eggs frozen at our local fertility center that we paid to ship to Syracuse. In the fall of 2020, when the whole world was upside down, we drove ten hours back and forth to New York for treatments chasing a final fragile hope. Our first round of IVF resulted in another chemical pregnancy—another flicker of life taken too soon. We were devastated but resolved to use all our eggs. We placed all our hope in God's hands, transferring our very last embryo. On April 22, 2021, we welcomed Violet Elliana (meaning "God answered") into our world, and our family was complete. And so that was the end. I never had to think about those nightmarish years we went through ever again, right? (Insert laughs.)

About a year after Violet was born, we took the whole family on a hike in the mountains of Maine. Even though it was summertime, the winds whipped and temps dropped to fifty degrees Fahrenheit. We bundled up in all the clothes we could find in our car and wandered out to the breath-taking summit. I walked over to a sign that said, "Not so Barren." The sign was in reference to Cadillac Mountain, which is known for growth despite its rocky granite slopes, uneven desert surfaces, and harsh weather conditions near its summit. "Cadillac Mountain may appear barren in places," the sign read, "but look closely and you will find pockets of alpine plants and clusters of stunted trees." I chuckled to myself as I shifted the weight of my little girl to my other hip.

Now with three children, born out of the grace of God through science, this is how I probably look to outsiders: *not so barren*. Sure, based on the views from the summit of my life, it looks that way. But many had no clue of the harsh seasons we had endured. They exclaim, "Wow, your hands are full!" And without a doubt, my family and friends probably breathed a sigh of relief now that I was "not so barren." It's all over. I should be over it, too, right? I hear the unspoken remarks: "Whew, we don't have to talk about that anymore. She got what she wanted. Chapter closed."

Not quite.

My body still suffers from the effects of endometriosis, and on its own, it will probably never produce a baby. The labels of "infertile" and "bereaved mother" never completely left me.

The tension of both privilege and responsibility in parenting through the lens of loss weighs heavy. And my heart will forever be marked by the transformation that happened through those barren years.

On Cadillac Mountain, there is life in a seemingly dead place. A flowering plant bursts forth from broken granite crevices all over the mountain. The whipping winds, torrential snow and ice, and low soil levels would suggest this mountain is far too harsh an environment to sustain any life. And yet, against all odds, life breaks forth, thriving. My heart used to be just like that mountain. Cold, stripped bare by the storms of loss and disappointment. There was no soil of hope left. But God burst through in the weathered places and I began to grow trust and hope where my heart was barren. A false god I had created crumbled to reveal the God who was always there, loving me and holding me that I had lost sight of. What was once fragile now shows evidence of His transformation in me, bringing new growth and beauty in the most unexpected of places. "What cracks our heart open more deeply to God's love is our loss of everything except His love. In our devastation, God welcomes us in" (Ortland, 2025, 33).

These stories are never easy to read or process, but I believe that, in sharing, we can build trust and see God's hand working. I pray that my story may strengthen yours and be the image of hope to look to in the valley. As we move through the next pages, I pray you feel that you can trust me with your heart on the road ahead while I lead you through stories of women in the Bible like us (or your loved one). We will look closely at these stories to see the transformation that took place in their hearts, both good and bad, as a result of their journeys. Along the way, I will give further details to my story as it relates to each of these women, I will share wisdom I learned from these women, and highlight some of the key lessons to help in the days ahead. I will also provide insight and advice for those in the wider circles of support trying to walk alongside to their loved ones.

I would like to close this chapter by asking that we take along an abundance of grace with us on this trip. While my story had redemption, that may not be the case for all who read this book. If this is you—know that you are seen, and your losses are deeply grieved by our heavenly Father. While I believe there is restoration in each of our stories, sometimes it does not come in ways we hope or expect. Even so, God promises He is with us every step of the way, and we can count on Him to be faithful. "Remember your word to your servant, for you have given me hope. My comfort in my suffering is this: Your promise preserves my life" (Psalm 119:49–50 NIV).

I also recognize our paths will likely have varying landscapes: different barriers, different diagnoses, emotional and financial factors, and different convictions. My own journey started nearly thirteen years ago, so it should be expected that standards have changed. Many states have mercifully passed bills which mandated insurance companies to provide fertility coverage. I will share with you to the best of my memory, detailed procedures, treatments, and experiences, but it should be noted that these are not meant to point you to a particular path or give medical advice. Rather, it is in my sharing that I hope to point you to how God was at work in each detail. And as we read, reflect, and explore together, my hope is you will see you are not alone on your journey. Even on the bad days. You are surrounded by God's love, by His grace, and by a sisterhood of women who walked this road thousands of years before us. Come, let's go together, for they have much to teach us.

[Author's recommendations: I encourage readers to review the Bible passages listed before reading the chapter to familiarize yourself with the stories in the Bible. For group study: Have each reader review Before We Start and My Story on their own and then start group discussion with Sarai.]

Sarai

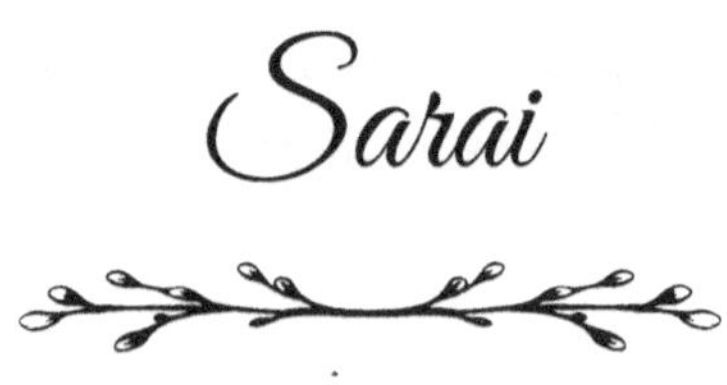

Chronologically, Sarai was the first woman in the Bible to experience infertility. Her story comes on the heels of several directives from God to fill the earth. From the first pages of Scripture, fruitfulness was a calling. Adam and Eve were called to fill the earth and subdue it (Genesis 1:28). After the flood, Noah received the same charge (Genesis 9:1). In light of these divine directives, infertility must have felt like a contradiction to God's plan. How very confusing and hurtful it must have been to not be able to fulfill this calling. I wonder how this affected Sarai's relationship with God. I wonder if she felt forgotten, cursed, or undervalued by Him.

While Sarai was conflicted about God's calling, Abram, her husband, was blessed to engage in regular intimate conversations with Him. God gave him a gift of divine promise, the Abrahamic covenant. The covenant was in three parts: that all nations would come through him, that his name would be great, and that he and all those in his family line would be blessed. But there were strings attached. Abram had to leave the only country he ever knew to move to an unknown land. And much of God's promises relied on the offspring Abram did not yet have. How do you trust in a promise that contradicts your current situation?

But Abram chose to be obedient; he left his childhood home and everything he knew. He traveled four hundred grueling miles with Sarai and his nephew, Lot, arriving in Shechem, Canaan. It was there that God appeared a second time likely in a theophany or a visible manifestation like an angel. He told Abram that He would give this land to his children. Even though God's plan made absolutely no sense to him, Abram responded by building an altar to worship and mark this moment of faith without sight.

More challenges came later as the "promised land" developed a famine. They detoured to Egypt hoping to find food instead of looking to God to provide where they were. The trouble didn't stop there. Once in Egypt, it became clear Sarai was in imminent danger of being abducted to Pharoah's harem as she was very attractive. It was common practice in those times for rulers to poach foreign wives and to kill their husbands. So when Pharaoh's henchmen came to take Sarai, Abram left her unprotected by lying and saying that she was his sister. He prioritized his protection over her safety. Left vulnerable, she was taken into Pharaoh's kingdom while Abram was treated with favor. He was gifted a multitude of livestock, servants, and goods.

I can only imagine at this point Sarai felt not only terrified but abandoned by her husband and God. Her husband deeply betrayed her and also benefited from the betrayal. It was clear that he did not trust God's promise of a prosperous future because he feared death so much he put her life in danger. But God stepped in. He inflicted diseases on Pharaoh, who released Sarai and ordered Abram and her out of Egypt. As they walked out of Pharaoh's palace, I wonder how the conversation went. Abram—stumbling over his words, sheepish and guilty. Sarai likely silent, but relieved and deeply wounded. Yet God had not left her. He swooped in as her rescuer, in place of her husband. God saw and continued to push His promise forward, even in the midst of Abram's unfaithfulness.

Abram chose to go back to the land where he last built an altar to the Lord to regain his footing. When they arrived, he and Lot split ways as the land could no longer support them both. Since Lot was his only other living relative, Abram's future grew more uncertain because he still had no children to call his own. God returned, confirming this land would belong to Abram's children who would be as numerous as the dust of the earth. Well, that sounds nice, but when? How? Still, we can see some of the fruits of God's promises peeking through as God was faithful to grow Abram's possessions and land.

God also proved His faithfulness as Abram grew in power and strength. He protected his family just like He said He would, and still, Abram had no children. So, God came to him in a vision, a third time to renew and provide new clarity on His promise.

> "Do not be afraid, Abram. I am your shield, your very great reward."
>
> But Abram said, "Sovereign LORD, what can you give me since I remain childless and the one who will inherit my estate is Eliezer of Damascus?" And Abram said, "You have given me no children; so a servant in my household will be my heir."
>
> Then the word of the Lord came to him: "This man will not be your heir, but a son who is your own flesh and blood will be your heir." He took him outside and said, "Look up at the sky and count the stars—if indeed you can count them." Then he said to him, "So shall your offspring be."
>
> Abram believed the LORD, and he credited it to him as righteousness.
>
> Genesis 15:1–6 NIV

What tender and powerful words God poured out to Abram. "I am your shield, your very great reward" (Genesis 15:1 NIV). God kept showing up faithfully for Abram when he needed it most, even after his mistakes. This time He reminded Abram *who He was*. And that was exactly what Abram needed to hear. He needed to know I AM, the LORD, Yahweh was on his side. Abram needed a shield to protect him from the enemies surrounding him. His men had just defeated an army of four kingdoms defending his wayward nephew, Lot, and there was threat of retaliation. And yet, amid an all-out war, Abram was still distracted by his lack, reminding the Lord He still needed to make good on this promise of a son.

Abram cried out to God, "Wait, You promised me all of these things, but who's going to inherit this wealth and name that You blessed me with?" He was discouraged. He was resigned to pass everything on to his servant as was custom for families with no children in those days. But God said, "a son who is your own flesh and blood will be your heir"(Genesis 15:4 NIV). This was good clarifying information because, after all this time, Abram probably couldn't help but look for another strategy.

God knew Abram needed something more tangible to hold onto, and so the Creator of the universe took him outside and showed him the stars of the sky. He said, "So shall your offspring be" (Genesis 15:4 NIV). Seeing the countless stars in the unveiled sky assured Abram the God of the heavens was capable. He believed God could be trusted and it was accounted to him as righteousness. This accounting to him as righteousness business was a monumental moment that transcends to our current day. He had faith, but now he was clothed in God's righteousness. This was salvation by grace through faith, long before Jesus had even entered the world. This moment should give us confidence that God had a plan for us from the beginning, that our righteousness would come from Jesus. Romans 4:19–24 (NIV) tells us:

> Without weakening in his faith, he faced the fact that his body was as good as dead—since he was about a hundred years old—and that Sarah's womb was also dead. Yet he did not waver through unbelief regarding the promise of God, but was strengthened in his faith and gave glory to God, being fully persuaded that God had power to do what he promised. This is why "it was credited to him as righteousness." The words "it was credited to him" were not written for him alone, but also for us.

But also for us. This promise is as much for you and me, friend, as it was for Abram. Are you willing to believe? Or are God's promises starting to feel empty to you? Ask God to reveal the promises He has already fulfilled in your life. Look back to the cross. Look at the small ways He's meeting your needs. Write them down, and if you can, carry them with you because the devil will always show up with his baggage of doubt. Do you need a reminder? Look at the stars, friend. His righteousness, His trustworthiness is all there. That promise is still for us. Marvel at His creation. Ask him to show you *who He is*. He will. He was faithful to His promises for Abram and Sarai and He will be faithful to His promises to you.

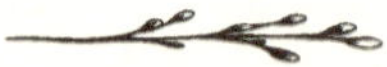

On my journey, there were so many nights I, like Abram, struggled to see God's plan. I often found peace in taking long walks at night with my sweet but anxious Labrador, Maizey. I can't recommend them enough. Maybe it's the silence, allowing your thoughts to wander, maybe it's necessary meditation. I enjoyed my late-night walks, as the dead of night provided the much-needed security of being alone. Sometimes I cried out to the Lord, and other times I held a stony silence between us.

In the days following Christmas, I set out for my usual night walk. After enduring a holiday season known to be magical for little ones, I found my arms and heart empty. Advent, an expectant season filled with hope, had once again left me wanting. For those of you who may be trying to support a loved one, remember that Christmas can be a particularly difficult time, as it serves as a timestamp for unmet expectations. I was angry, tired, and emotionally poured out from congregating with friends and family. All their questions and well-meaning reassurances had exhausted me.

"What is happening?"

"Have you tried …"

"Just give it time."

Maizey and I plodded through the icy snow, trying not to slip. I took in deep, angry breaths of cold air, watching the steam dissipate in the starry sky as I exhaled. Tears slipped down my face as I quietly grieved the lack of family we so desperately wanted. Brent and I had both come from bigger families with three kids each. No one in my immediate circles understood what we were going through. We, like many couples, did not expect to wait for years to have a baby. It seemed most of those around us had no issues growing their families. That night, I had nothing to bring to the Lord but my frustration, deep sadness, and lament. I was on the brink of giving up. I was exhausted with this story, and I had begun to think everything was not going to work out. Similar to Abram, I kept losing hope. Every holiday was a reminder that we didn't have children, and it became harder and harder to find joy.

It was that walk when something changed. Suddenly I deeply felt the Holy Spirit interceding for me in a way I had not before. Something moved deep inside of me like a sharp exhale. In that moment, God met me. Enveloped in the dark, cold air, something stopped me in my tracks. I stood completely still as though I was stopped in front of a brick wall. Maizey looked at me strangely but resigned to lie down while all this got worked out. My eyes squinted to see what was happening, but there was nothing to see but the velvety night sky. My skin tingled, goosebumps forming. It was almost as though I felt the Lord nose to nose with me, so close, so palpable. I struggled to put words to the sensation I felt, but I knew the Lord had passed me by. Relief and peace washed over me as two of my favorite Bible verses welled up in my heart: "Fear not, for I am with you; be not dismayed, [Heather], for I am your God; I will strengthen you, I will help you, I will uphold you with my righteous right hand" (Isaiah 41:10 ESV). "Therefore we do not lose heart. Though outwardly we are wasting away, yet inwardly we are being renewed day by day. For our light and momentary troubles are achieving for us an eternal glory that far outweighs them all. So we fix our eyes not on what is seen, but on what is unseen, since what is seen is temporary, but what is unseen is eternal" (2 Corinthians 4:16–18 NIV).

I stood still in quiet amazement as sparkly little snowflakes swirled around me. I looked up at the night sky, not knowing what happened to me and in me. But I was sure the presence of the Lord had encircled me. For the rest of the walk, Christmas lights seemed brighter, stars twinkled a little twinklier. I had no choice but to accept the awe of His presence and soak in the peace that passed understanding.

Friend, lift your eyes to the stars. The Creator of the universe intercedes for you.

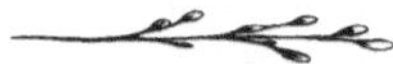

Some years after Abram entered into this covenant with God, Sarai formulated her own plan for how to work out the child-bearing portion of the promise, as it was not happening through her. "See now, the Lord has prevented me from bearing *children*" (Genesis 16:2 NASB). Not us, not Abram. Me. These words seem so matter of fact.

If I were Sarai, I probably would have phrased it as a question. *Why has the Lord kept me from bearing children?* But she's not asking that question; she's just stating a fact. *See now,* she says. *See now* points a finger. *See now* is definitive. She had given up on a multitude of unanswered prayers. She had come to a conclusion. This promise was for Abram, not her. She was the barrier, and she was looking for another solution to move the plan forward. While God was showering love and promises over Abram, she believed God was holding them back from her. And I can see why. God hadn't told her that she would be the mother of nations yet. That would come later, and it's clear from her actions that she didn't know it.

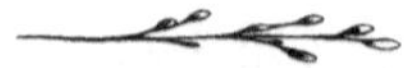

The days of ongoing testing, enduring doctors' visits, multiple blood tests, ultrasounds, contrast studies, biopsies, pills, and shots are hard to erase from my memory.

"It all looks normal."

"Unexplained infertility."

"It will happen, give it more time."

Months and months and months of increasing heartache and doubt. Deep inside, a voice whispered, *It's you. It's your fault. This promise is not for you. You don't deserve it.*

Sometimes, the thoughts got even darker. *This is because of your sin. God is withholding a baby from you because of your past.*

And these poisonous thoughts weren't just coming from the dark corners in my own soul. Sometimes, they were said to me by the people in my life.

"Have you gone before the Lord and confessed?"

"Is there anything in your heart that God would not want?"

"Why do you think God is doing this to you?"

"Is this a punishment?"

My heart was desperate for a solution. I wanted there to be an answer, a reason for my suffering. I allowed these thoughts to linger for far too long. My mind drifted back to repented sins from years ago. I had cracked the door, and shame crept in. The forms I filled out at the fertility office asked the damning questions for me: "How many sexual partners have you had?" "Have you taken any medication that would prevent your fertility?" "Is there a medical reason for why you might not be able to get pregnant?"

I don't know why I even needed to answer these questions; multiple blood tests would confirm whether I checked those boxes truthfully.

The thing is, friends, we know there is a distinction between suffering and consequences of sin. Suffering does not equal wrongdoing. Suffering comes with the reality of living in a broken world. And we live in a world that groans with those pains of labor as it suffers the weight of sin (Romans 8:22). Infertility is the echo of those groans. Brokenness followed humanity out of Eden, bending us toward rebellion, which comes with consequences. For some of us, rebellion showed up as choices born out of loneliness, and longing for love. Even these shortcomings are not too far from grace. There is freedom in repentance, and God removes those transgressions as far as the east is from the west (Psalm 103:12). Do not let the deceiver wield his weak power by bringing up old sin where you have been set free.

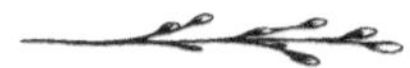

Let's return to Abram and Sarai. Sarai, believing she was excluded from the covenant and responsible for their child-lessness, sought out a new solution that would speed up their family-building. Can we blame her for wanting to rush to the happy ending? She decided to work out God's promise in Hagar. "Perhaps I can build a family through her" (Genesis 16:2 NIV). Sarai believed she could control God's promise. Hagar was an Egyptian maidservant who was likely given to Abram as a gift during the "she is my sister" incident. Remember, Pharaoh had shown favor to Abram in the form of servants. Hagar had come into this family because of Abram's deceit, and the ripple effect of sin continued.

The version of surrogacy Sarai was offering was in direct opposition to God's purpose for marriage, but it was a common Near Eastern practice. Sarai thought she was helping usher in the promises of God, but her solution tragically led to more sin and further desecration of her marriage.

Disappointingly, Abram agreed to Sarai's suggestion and slept with Hagar. She became pregnant and bore a son whom she named Ishmael. Sarai then became jealous of Hagar and mistreated her, leading to increased conflicts between them, and ultimately, Hagar and Ishmael went on the run. Yet we see God's plans superseding all others, including Sarai's. Even in this misguided path, He would build His earthly kingdom through both Ishmael and the soon-to-be conceived child of Abram and Sarai.

We have all done some version of this. I know I have. God leads us to a promise that hasn't quite unfolded yet, and we say, "No problem, God. I'll finish this up for You and You can come along with me." I'm a doer. I like to get things done quickly and efficiently. I like a plan, and I like control. I like to know what the next step is. Waiting is not something that bodes well with me. Do you, too, find yourself reaching for control when things get messy?

For me, this moment was highlighted during our second round of IVF after our first miscarriage. After that pregnancy loss, something in me felt unfinished. I had grasped something in my heart, a dream in my mind, that felt like it was stolen from me. And now my heart couldn't forget that there was a chance I could be blessed with a third child. Once that thought took root, I couldn't shake it. Something in me had to prove that death was not the end of my journey, at any cost. But month after month, heartache after heartache, there was no sign of hope. After sixteen months of trying naturally, we decided to pursue another round of IVF. We knew the process well and what was necessary. I opted to repeat surgery prior to IVF to remove any possible inflammatory tissue from my pelvis that might be preventing me from getting pregnant. "Surely this will work," my doctor told me, and I told myself.

My bruised abdomen showed the signs of beatings that my body had taken from surgery. My boys winced, pointing at my bruised belly, and said, "Mama ... owie." In addition to my frayed nerves of wondering if this cycle would work, our finances hemorrhaged under the weight of medication bills, doctor visits, ultrasounds, and procedures. I was under weight-lifting restrictions, so I couldn't pick up my sweet toddlers for weeks. It broke me that I couldn't fill my arms with them. The ones I had waited so long for. They would lift their little chubby hands, waving to me, saying, "Mama! Mama!" My heart was crushed to not lift them, but I knew I had to give this treatment my all. Everything had to be done the right way, the only way we knew. The limitations reached my spiritual and emotional life as well. My heart showed signs of hardening, as I became guarded. I prayed less, I sought wisdom from online medical research, online forums, and less frequently on my knees.

"I'm so sorry, Mrs. LaVigne, your beta HCG level is 13. We will perform serial lab testing to see if this pregnancy sticks, but you need to prepare for the possibility of a chemical pregnancy." It is important to note that healthy pregnancies most often produce beta HCG blood levels greater than 20. Two days later, my HCG levels dropped to 3, and my discouragement dropped even lower. Something that was once alive died in me all over again.

We happened to be making a twenty-two-hour drive in a cramped car to Florida from Michigan when we were burdened with this grief. I don't think there is ever a perfect situation in which to get this news, but I'm confident this was the least desirable. This was the first time I was prescribed serial testing to determine if my pregnancy was viable.

Let me explain a bit more about serial testing as it may not be familiar to most, especially for those supporting a loved one. A woman with low beta HCG levels will need to return to a lab or clinic for blood testing every two to three days. The expectation is that either the level goes up or down. If the number goes down, it means she has had a chemical pregnancy and inevitably will lose this pregnancy. The blood must be redrawn until it reaches zero to ensure the hormone levels have returned to normal, "not pregnant" levels. If the numbers go up, they must be carefully checked every few days to ensure the embryo is growing, as it is deemed at risk. This process of frequent blood draws is called serial testing or blood work purgatory, as I commonly referred to it.

Going through serial testing to determine whether you are maintaining a pregnancy or miscarrying is one of the most anxiety-producing, gut-wrenching waiting times in one's life. Losing a pregnancy following serial testing is devastating. The baby you worked so hard for has now passed away. You are either waiting to pass this baby out of your womb or have begun to pass it. It's like a ticking time bomb. And if that's not enough, you must roll up your sleeve for another poke to confirm something you already know: Your baby has died. Your body has expelled something that was meant to grow. This must be done to confirm the hormones have left the body in preparation for the next cycle. The worst part? You have to sit in waiting rooms next to women with healthy pregnancies. It is one of the most demoralizing experiences, a walk of shame of sorts, passing by all the growing bellies, feeling like a failure.

It can be hard to know how to support your loved one in this tenuous situation. Sometimes that support is going to look different day to day. Expect to see swings in emotion, depression, and irritability. If someone you love is going through serial testing, try to remember the painful passages that must be walked through and keep in mind that these can truly be some of the darkest days your loved one will experience. Consider offering to go to the lab with them. Check in, but be sensitive about asking details.

Trapped in a car on a road trip for two days, I waited for my period with dread. My young sons blissfully had no idea the tragedy our family had just suffered. A recent discovery of the joy of McDonald's caused them to shriek anytime they saw those massive golden arches from the highway. They labeled it "hotta lotta" in their own twin language and begged for it any time the "M" could be spotted. We just stayed on the highway, staring blankly at the road ahead. Brent and I sat in silence for much of that drive. He was lost for what to say and burdened with his own grief and anxieties. I remained quiet until the next call or text came through from a friend or family member who had prayed for a different answer. The stressors soared even higher when the follow-up call came from my reproductive endocrinologist. She told me she was concerned there may be an underlying auto-immune disorder causing my miscarriages, since this was my second loss.

"I would recommend a lupus workup," she told me. My heart sank as I wound the car through the mountains of Kentucky. I already had one chronic disease, and my thoughts were over-whelmed with the idea of having another, never mind the glaring fact that my body was still unable to do what it was created to do.

"Do you want to try IVF again?" she asked.

"I can't!" I angrily blurted out at her, "I can't do this anymore, emotionally, financially…"

"I understand. Call us if you need us."

Like that, the line went dead. A heavy cloak of clouds rolled over our car, and tiny raindrops fell on our windshield. Tears streamed down my face as I worried about the cost this ongoing nightmare had on my body, our finances, and our stability.

Sarah

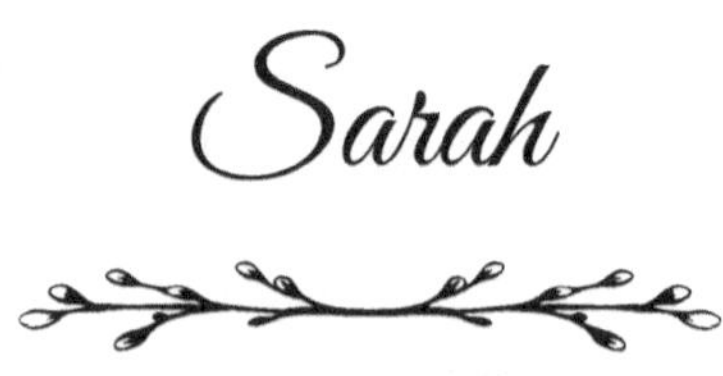

This chapter is not about a new biblical character but, rather, highlights her divine name change from Sarai to Sarah. Not only does she receive a name change, but she also gets a role change as well. The long-awaited moment is here when we see her become a mother. When Sarai was eighty-nine years old, and Abram was ninety-nine years old, God returned once more to reaffirm His promise, and the covenantal promise grew.

God renamed Abram "Abraham," meaning "father of many nations." Abram had meant "father of many," which was a painful irony because Abram was still the father of none. The meanings of these names showed God was doubling down on His promise, which was still pending. Sarai was to be Sarah, which meant, "the mother of nations, princess to all." Sarai, at its Jewish root meant, "my princess or princess to one family" (Eames 2022). This confirmation showed Sarai was indeed an integral part of the covenant, not a bystander or plan B, but chosen from the beginning and always had been. A son would be given through her. In fact, kings of nations would come from her. No surrogacy needed.

But expansion of the covenant came with new strings attached—a commitment to being faithful and obedient to God, which meant that Abraham and his entire household must be circumcised. This act signified the cutting away of their self-reliance and was a sign that their confidence was in God rather than their own flesh. God's promise came at a cost to all of them. They had to be dependent and obedient.

Deciding to follow through on their recommended name change also required a response from Abraham and Sarah. They had to take hold of God's promise by agreeing to identify differently. The essence of who they were had to change. They had to tell all their friends and family to refer to them with their new names and explain that God had initiated that change. Can you even imagine? One day, my name is Heather, and the next day, I'm calling my mom and telling her I changed the name she so lovingly gave me to Harriet. I can feel her bewildered response… "Um…why?" They would have to explain that God was going to do a new thing. They had to be confident He would come through. This promise was no longer private; it was public. Abraham and Sarah had followed through, and it was up to God to come through on this promise of a child.

The LORD appeared to Abraham near the great trees of Mamre while he was sitting at the entrance to his tent in the heat of the day. Abraham looked up and saw three men standing nearby. When he saw them, he hurried from the entrance of his tent to meet them and bowed low to the ground. […]"

"Where is your wife, Sarah?" they asked him.

"There in the tent," he said.

Then one of them said, "I will surely return to you about this time next year, and Sarah, your wife, will have a son."

Now Sarah was listening at the entrance to the tent, which was behind him. […] Sarah laughed to herself as she thought, "After I am worn out and my lord is old, will I now have this pleasure?"

> Then the LORD said to Abraham, "Why did Sarah laugh and say, 'Will I really have a child, now that I am old?' Is anything too hard for the LORD? I will return to you at the appointed time next year, and Sarah will have a son."
>
> Genesis 18:1–2, 9–10, 12 NIV

Soon after the name change, three men came to Sarah and Abraham's home to provide another confirmation of God's promise. The men represented God or a Christophany appearing to Abraham at his tent. They came with an important message and a timeline. In the next year, Sarah would have her baby. After lifelong infertility, it was finally her turn. When she said, "Will I now have this pleasure?" I wonder if what she meant was, "God, are you sure about your timing?" Was this finally going to happen? Can you even imagine what it was like to think about having a baby in the next year…at nearly ninety years old? When I read this passage, I laugh. *Sister, I don't blame you. I wouldn't have the strength to believe it either.*

A quarter of a century had passed since God first spoke of the covenantal promise. Abraham and Sarah had endured decades of waiting and unknowns of why they couldn't conceive. They had carried the stress associated with not being able to grow their family, and they feared the loss of their family legacy. Hagar and Ishmael had long been banished, leaving a wounded heritage. Sarah had spent years surrounded by pregnant bellies and small children. Now advanced in age, she may have been relieved to have outgrown the fertile stages of life, but likely wistfully watched on as families grew with grandchildren, and hers did not. She must have thought, "Will I now have this pleasure? Really God? You're going to do this now? Now, long after menopause, when I've already lost most of my good years, when my body is worn out. Next year, really?" I wonder if she couldn't help but doubt His promise.

When I unexpectedly became pregnant on my own after years of treatments and procedures, I had no idea what to do. I called all my friends and asked, "What do you do after you see a positive sign on the pee stick?" This was all foreign to me. I was familiar with blood tests, ovulation kits, invasive ultrasounds, and careful measurements. Peeing on a stick seemed very unreliable. Brent and I were stunned, scared, and elated to see a positive test that was not assisted by science. *Would I now have this pleasure? Was God's timing right?*

A few weeks later, we went to the ultrasound appointment with our boys to celebrate this new, unexpected, miraculous life. We all crowded in the tiny, dimly lit room, only to see a vacant black circle in my uterus reflected on the monitor. No heartbeat, no fetal pole, no signs of life.

"This looks like a case of a blighted ovum," said the technician. "Your fertilized egg implanted in the uterus, but it failed to develop." Inside, my whole being screamed at God, *Why would You do this to me?* My nearly one-year-old boys babbled away in the arms of my husband next to me as we silently stared at the screen.

"Get them out," I murmured. He nodded, silently backing out of the room as Dr LG came in.

I half-listened to the doctor as I steeled myself for the conversations that would come next.

"You can take a pill or just let it pass naturally."

"It will be uncomfortable, but you are strong and healthy. You can do it."

"I'm so sorry."

"These happen all the time. You could still have a healthy pregnancy."

"This is a good thing. Maybe your body can do it on its own now."

I never even considered that I might be able to experience the joy of another pregnancy, never mind a natural one. *Why must I endure a new layer of pain in addition to the pain the prior years of childlessness had produced?* We thought our valley was over. My hope continued to erode over the next few weeks as my body was unable to completely pass the miscarriage on its own. I went on to take two rounds of Misoprostol (medication used to expel pregnancy tissue), causing extreme illness. Unfortunately, even that didn't work, and I went on to need a D&C several months later. The entire joy of pregnancy had been stripped from me. Everything felt medicalized and doomed to fail. Both my heart and my body were broken. Like Sarah, my faith grew thin as I started to doubt God's promises.

The trials continued for Sarah and Abraham. They moved to Gerar, a new area of their promised land that neighbored an enemy, the Philistines. Abraham, again, told the lie that Sarah was his sister because he feared he would be killed when they attempted to take her. Did he learn nothing from before? (Note: Sarah had clearly aged well as she was coming into her nineties and continued to attract kings far and wide).

Sarah indeed was captured and taken into the Philistine king's household. But before anything happened, God came to the king in a dream, with a warning that Sarah was a married woman and threatened death over his kingdom if she wasn't returned. King Abimelech called Abraham in for questioning and Abraham weakly defended himself, explaining that Sarah was his half-sister (which wasn't uncommon in those times), but was also truthfully his wife. Sarah was returned along with many gifts (sheep, cattle, servants, land, and silver) as penance for wife-stealing.

You might scratch your head, wondering why King Abimelech would give gifts *after* he gave Sarah back. Wasn't giving Sarah back enough? King Abimelech was motivated to make things right because after Sarah arrived, his household had been afflicted with a plague that God told him only Abraham could heal with prayer. So, Abraham prayed, and God healed Abimelech, his wife, and his female slaves. Healed of what, you ask? The curse of infertility. The Lord had kept every female from childbearing while Sarah was in Abimelech's household, and it was Abraham's prayers that healed them.

Whoa… whoa…whoa… Let's back up. Abraham and Sarah were still waiting on God to provide them with their promised baby. God had told them this would happen in the next year.

While it had been years since the first promise of a baby, we are now working with a God-given timeline. The same lie was told by Abraham to protect himself because his wife was too beautiful. Sarah, again, was basically trafficked. She went into that household and *boom*, no one could get pregnant. She was given back to her rightful husband, who prayed for the king's household, and magically, everyone started getting pregnant again. Well, everyone except Sarah.

Can you even imagine? You become an infertility blast zone to everyone around you. Contagious to all who come into contact. Until everyone was healed by your husband's prayer. But God didn't answer any of those prayers for you yet. Ouch.

I believe God was showing Abraham and Sarah, "Look at what I can do through and around you. Let go. I am in control." I cannot even begin to imagine how much that stung for them. The very thing they desperately desired and struggled to believe would happen was quickly restored and given to everyone but them, both as a reminder and a consequence of their actions.

This story brings back familiar emotions during a time when I was leading women's Bible studies. I was relatively new to this conservative community of women, which, unbeknownst to me, held high regard for family building and family support—two things I was lacking in. I joined as a member a year earlier, and I felt the Lord leading me to step into leadership. I was cautious about sharing what I was going through for a lot of reasons, but mostly because my life experience felt so different from everyone else's.

While everyone celebrated new (and often accidental) life on a cyclical basis, I regularly grieved the death of a dream. In the next year of leadership, over half of the group of women I was shepherding announced they were pregnant. I was baffled that, while I was obedient to the Lord and infertile, everyone around me seemed to be getting what I desired so badly. What is it about women's Bible studies and proliferative pregnancies? Maybe it's the appeal of a break from crabby toddlers, hot coffee, and coveted silence, but these Bible studies seem to be a microcosm of gestating women. While the fault was none of theirs, I found myself triggered on a weekly basis.

In this community, it wasn't uncommon to ask incredibly personal questions about family planning. Can we talk about how uncomfortable it is to share about how you can't have a baby, particularly in a circle that includes several pregnant women?

In a season of miscarriages, I was silently struggling just to make it through the day. One afternoon after Bible study, a woman pulled me aside and shared with me that she had been surprised to learn her daughter was expecting, and it was an unplanned pregnancy. She was overcome with joy that the baby would be born just in time for Christmas. She leaned in closely and told me that she wished that I, too, could have a Christmas baby. It was all a bit too much. My mask began to crack. I gave her a quick hug, thanked her, and I ran to the bathroom to have a panic attack.

Over the course of my involvement in this Bible study, many well-meaning women asked me over and over and over again, "Are you expecting? When will you have another little one? Will you have more children?" There were many teas and potlucks where we gathered around covered tables, sharing our lives with one another. Giggles burst out when someone said there might be more children coming. There were laughs about the unexpected pregnancies that produced the happy toddlers running around the table. Shouts of joy rang out in response as a pregnancy announcement came from a nearby group. Everyone would crane their necks, eagerly awaiting the news. At one ladies' lunch, it became apparent that every woman around the table had five children except me. I offered, "Well, I have a set of twins?" From the outside, I probably looked uber-fertile, having had multiple children at once. My little curly headed miracles. Were they not enough? My heart sank, knowing I had indeed carried five children, but three of them hadn't made it to this side of heaven.

Only by the grace and strength of God did I make it through that season of life. I constantly waffled between resentment and fear of the next pregnancy announcement while dealing with the shame of infertility. However, this ongoing tension created a growing need for me to regularly rely on my Savior.

If you struggle like I did in social circles, can I encourage you to lean toward those who can best support you where you are and release yourself from obligations that may cause triggering during particularly sensitive seasons? If you are struggling, I'd like to offer you permission to kindly defer mom's Bible studies, MOPS (Mothers of Preschoolers), or similar groups. Looking back, I wish someone had given me permission to do so. It could have saved me a boatload of emotions. Consider searching out churches with support groups dedicated to infertility or find an online biblical community supporting women going through infertility and pregnancy loss that can support you.

It may also be necessary to put a gentle distance between you and a friend who is pregnant. Celebrate her as best you can but be honest with your feelings and capacity for pregnancy-related talk. Take stock of your conversations and who you converse with. This may mean you might keep to small talk only with that family member who has a propensity for asking the probing questions. Think about keeping a support person in the room with you at family parties in case you need a conversation "diverter." Sometimes this was my husband, other times it was a close friend. If you are a dear one supporting a friend struggling, volunteer to be this person. It's helpful to have practiced responses to avoid that deer-in-the-headlights moment like I had with my Bible study. Practice them in the mirror to ensure they feel natural but can quickly release you from a triggering moment.

If you are a supporter, kindly consider the small talk you keep in public circles. Instead of asking," How many kids do you have?" Consider saying," What does your family look like?" Avoid asking women of childbearing age if they have children and other personal questions involving family growing.

Finally, consider seeking counseling. I was supported for years by a woman who provided sharp wisdom and kind solace. There are many therapists who specialize in infertility and infant loss who may be integral on the road to healing. Don't wait until your next crisis to seek out help. Most importantly, bring it to the

Lord, my sweet friend. His hands are trustworthy to hold what you are carrying.

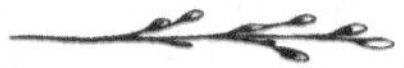

> Now the Lord was gracious to Sarah, as he said, and the Lord did for Sarah what he had promised. Sarah became pregnant and bore a son to Abraham in his old age, at the very time God had promised him. […] Sarah said, "God has brought me laughter and everyone who hears about this will laugh with me." And she added, "'Who would have said to Abraham that Sarah would nurse children? Yet I have borne him a son in his old age.'"

Genesis 21:1–2, 6–7 NIV

Here is the moment we all have been waiting for! The fulfillment of the long-awaited promise: a baby born to Sarah and Abraham. Abraham was 100. *One hundred.* Sarah was ninety years old. Talk about a miracle. And … it happened at the very time God had promised them. He had clearly reviewed His promise with Abraham five separate times. And guess what? He's true to His word and His timing. Sarah overflowed with gratefulness and joy. She said, "God has literally stunned me to the point of laughter, and everyone who hears about this will laugh with me."

I think we all know this type of laughter. When something takes you by complete surprise and you can't help but bust out a good belly laugh. She named her son Isaac, which means "he will laugh," or "one who rejoices." What an amazing miracle. God was gracious to Sarah, just as He said He would be. He can be counted on. Even more so, He is abundant in His care for us.

Abraham and Sarah, advanced in age, likely feared that they would run out of time, unable to live long enough to see Isaac grow. Luckily, that was not the case. God extended Sarah's life for thirty more years, giving her the gift of full motherhood. She enjoyed her sweet son, Isaac, long after she birthed him. Long after the skinned knees and awkward teen years. She walked alongside him, loving him, and counseling him until he grew into a man. And Isaac returned her love. The Bible says they had a very special relationship; Isaac deeply grieved her passing (Genesis 24:67). I have a feeling that if we asked Sarah, she would say it was all worth it. In time, sorrow was replaced with laughter. Waiting was sacred preparation, not punishment. The promise was greater than the pain.

Rebekah

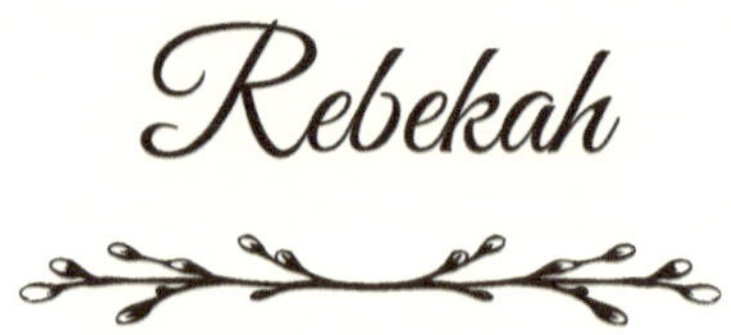

Genesis 24–25

Before we study Rebekah and Isaac's journey, let's get to know them a little better and travel back to how they met. I don't know about you, but I adore a good love story, and I believe it provides a broader context for us.

Isaac, the miracle baby of Abraham and Sarah, was to be the executor of all of Abraham's riches and wealth. At that time, the family lived in Canaan, surrounded by people who worshipped other gods. It was of critical importance that Isaac's wife come from Abraham's family line to preserve the covenant and family lineage. So, Abraham sent his senior servant (scholars assume this was Eliezer, the servant that would have been his heir had Isaac not been born) twelve hundred miles on camels loaded up with gifts for the family of the bride-to-be. What a loyal servant to make this grueling journey of epic importance.

After weeks of travel, he came into the city of Nahor. It was around evening time, when women routinely went out to draw water for their homes. Before he entered near a watering hole, Abraham's servant prayed to God to lead him to the right woman. He asked for a specific sign to identify the chosen woman for Isaac: She would provide water to him and offer to water his camels as well.

Before he even finished the prayer, he saw Rebekah with a jar on her shoulder going to the spring. When she came up, he asked for a drink, and she immediately gave it to him. Then, she offered to water his camels as well, completely unaware that her actions confirmed she was the one God had chosen for Isaac. She was so kindhearted, she actually hurried to carry the water jars to the animals and she made sure every one of them drank as much as they wanted. The servant watched her closely, knowing she was the one God had chosen. He gifted her with jewelry and asked to be taken before her family.

Upon arriving at her home, the servant explained the true purpose of his trip and how Rebekah had been confirmed by the Lord. The family agreed to the marriage arrangement, but asked that they wait to leave for ten days. The servant declined their request, saying he did not wish to be detained from his master further. It fell to Rebekah to make the final decision, and she agreed to go with him without delay. She left her family never to see them again, only to travel to an unknown place to marry a man she had never met. How's that for trust? Her family sent her off with a special blessing, wishing her abundant fertility and prosperity. And off they went on the weeks-long trip to meet her soon-to-be groom.

When Rebekah and the servant arrived in Negev (Southern Israel), Isaac was in the fields meditating on the Lord. Cue the love song music swirling in the background; enter Rebekah to the scene. As the story goes, they couldn't peel their eyes off each other, as if they had known one another for a lifetime. This is divine matchmaking. Abraham's servant caught up and regaled Isaac with the story of the Lord's provision and guidance in his securement of this stunningly beautiful woman. Isaac took Rebekah to his late mother's tent and married her, right then and there. The Bible says he deeply loved her and found solace in his grief over the loss of his mother in their newfound love.

So, what could go wrong? A match *literally* made in heaven. Yes and no. The same struggles that plagued their parents also plagued them: They became the second generation in a row to experience infertility. Why would God make a covenant rooted in fruitfulness with couples whom He had allowed to be infertile? In our Savior's greater wisdom, He chose to grow their hearts in faith and reliance, rather than their family number. Growing their family would come later.

For the first twenty years of their marriage, Isaac and Rebekah were unable to conceive. Isaac desperately prayed on behalf of his wife. And this must have been some superpower intercessory prayer. Because God showed up, not with one blessing, but with two: Rebekah became pregnant with twins.

One day, before any of my children were born, a dear friend of mine and I walked a familiar dusty path around Reeds Lake in East Grand Rapids. It was exactly five miles, and we walked it several times a week. We had reached the point of the walk where she usually starts asking me the tough questions, because that's what good friends do.

"Are you guys okay?" she asked. "You and Brent?"

We had recently failed another reproductive treatment, IUI (Intrauterine Insemination, a treatment where sperm is put directly in the uterus at the time of ovulation). As the fertility treatments became more complex, it became harder to manage the pressures of making it all work—the timed appointments, medication coordination, and the heaviest weight of our dashed expectations. Much of our life revolved around the next treatment or workup that needed to be done. I thought about it a bit and told her the truth.

"Not so good." I expressed my fears that this monster was taking over our lives and our hearts. She urged me to listen to the Lord and my body and consider a reset.

By then, I needed to be asked those hard questions, and I needed someone that was brave enough to ask them. I'd recently heard that infertile couples were three times as likely to divorce, and I was worried for us. My friend Lisa, whom I met through the RESOLVE support group, is one of those tragedies. Her story was much like mine, having gone years failing therapies and losing hope. She and her husband had saved up all their pennies for IVF. When she finally was able to afford the procedure, she did get pregnant, but she went on to lose her son Jeffrey at twenty weeks gestation.

An invasive bacteria took his life while he was in her womb. She not only lost him while he was still in her womb, but she also had to deliver him into the world asleep. I was mentally undone by this death and what she had been through. She invited me into her home to sit with her, and she shared his pictures with me. I stared at the little hands and feet. His not fully-formed little body. I took in the images of her and her husband holding Jeffrey, racked with grief and shock. I held the little booties that held his tiny feet. I hugged her and listened as she told me each detail of what happened.

There is rarely a time that I am not inspired by Lisa's persevering faith. She prioritizes Jesus first and family second, without hesitation or distractions. On so many occasions, she'd encouraged me to trust in the Lord and lean on His understanding when life threw curveballs. She has endured so many curveballs of her own, and yet she faithfully follows after her Savior.

The great grief of the loss of their son, their infertility journey, along with many other factors, sadly drove her marriage into a painful end. She is another friend willing to speak pointedly to me when I need it most. She often reminds me that I am blessed to not be one of the divorce data points and encourages me to look for grateful moments in my marriage.

A romantic love story is not enough to preserve a marriage when the valley comes. Even a match made in heaven is no match for infertility. Isaac and Rebekah needed God's help to open her womb. And in this case, Rebekah first needed Isaac to intercede in prayer for her. She was honest about her anxiety and pleaded with her husband to provide support. Prayer was the lynchpin that secured their marriage.

Do you and your husband pray together? Have you asked your husband to intercede for your broken womb? Friends, these are some of the most intimate, soul-searching prayers when the two of you can come together and pray to the Father who holds the answers. I implore you to start if you haven't already. Putting God in the center of this struggle is the most productive and protective thing you can do for your marriage.

In my own journey, there have been times when I have siloed myself in my own emotions and it's gotten me absolutely nowhere. Separation left me feeling hollow and irritable.

We disagreed with one another for an extended season about whether to complete another round of IVF. In therapy, Brent admitted that he was fearful for my life. He knew that I was strong, but the steady waves of disappointment were relentless. Every pregnancy ended in complications. He felt helpless watching the physical and emotional devastation due to the loss of our pregnancies. In his great love and protection for me, he feared we would not survive another heartbreak. He struggles with vulnerability as most men do, so this honesty was critical for our connection.

We are strongest in our marriage when we are transparent with ourselves and each other. We had to spend time internally assessing how we were feeling and admitting that out loud to each other. After being on a fertility treatment conveyor belt for years, I had lost track of what it was to internally process my feelings. It had become apparent that I was stuffing my grief when my NaPro doctor, after reviewing my history, gently pointed out that these miscarriages were real deaths I had experienced.

She paused to ask if I was okay. No one had asked me that before in any of my medical assessments. It was just a number to many specialists I had seen before. While I struggled to respond, she peered at me over my Creighton charts and asked poignantly if self care had been part of my past treatment? I realized the answer was a resounding "No."

In pushing forward, I had left parts of my own soul behind. I had to say many things out loud that would make many Christians shift in their seats: that I was deeply resentful toward God and had even turned toward Him in hatred; that I could no longer bring myself to open a Bible and read His Word; that I no longer prayed, yet still led women's groups; and that I no longer knew whether I could believe the theology I studied each week. I was lost. The entire life I had built in faith had crumbled and I had nowhere to go.

Admitting my soul's ache was incredibly hard for me, and it was even harder for my husband. We spent time together *and* separately processing the tragedies that rolled over our marriage. We sipped coffee and shared our hearts with trusted confidants. We took long walks and even longer drives, taking in the views of the beauty of creation. Our best talks were in the car, shoulder to shoulder, rather than face to face (less confrontational).

Once we could put honest words to the ache in our souls, we could do something with them. My pastor's wife sent a copy of "Dark Clouds, Deep Mercy" to my mailbox when I refused to leave the confines of my home. Mark Vroegop powerfully and gently put words to the groans my soul couldn't. We brought our ravage of emotions and complaints to God. We brought the hard questions. We brought our accusations. And guess what? God was not surprised by them. The more we brought, the more we felt a sense of release. God showed me He was more than capable to handle them and our grief. My hard heart broke and I started to pray the prayer that Mark prayed, "Lord, I trust in You to keep me trusting" (Vroegop, 2019, 85). Lament ushered me into a space for learning more about who He was and how to trust Him with my wounding. Lament shows our great need for Jesus who will one day come and make all things right in our incredibly broken world.

If you are looking for a resource for lament, look no further than the book of Psalms. The Psalms contains David's laments to the Lord in seemingly hopeless circumstances. Lamenting allowed us to release our fears, pain, and injustices to the Lord. If we do not lament, we hold it all in. In lament, we posture ourselves toward God, crying out to Him in prayer, believing that our relationship with Him will deepen in spite of our circumstances. Here are three of my favorite Psalms for lament:

> I cried out to God for help; I cried out to God to hear me. When I was in distress, I sought the Lord; at night I stretched out untiring hands, and I would not be comforted. I remembered you, God, and I groaned; I meditated and my spirit grew faint. You kept my eyes from closing; I was too troubled to speak. […] Will the Lord reject forever? Will he never show his favor again? Has his unfailing love vanished forever? Has his promise failed for all time? Has God forgotten to be merciful? Has he in his anger withheld his compassion? Then I thought, "To this I will appeal:

the years when the Most High stretched out his right hand. I will remember the deeds of the LORD; yes I will remember your miracles of long ago. I will consider all your works and meditate on all your mighty deeds."

Psalm 77:1–4, 7–12 NIV

My soul is deep in anguish. How long, LORD, how long? Turn, LORD, and deliver me; save me because of your unfailing love.

Psalm 6:3–4 NIV

How long, LORD? Will you forget me forever? How long will you hide your face from me? How long must I wrestle with my thoughts and day after day have sorrow in my heart? How long will my enemy triumph over me? Look on me and answer, LORD my God. Give light to my eyes, or I will sleep in death, and my enemy will say," I have overcome him," and my foes will rejoice when I fall. But I trust in your unfailing love; my heart rejoices in your salvation. I will sing the LORD's praise, for he has been good to me.

Psalm 13 NIV

If you are walking in the dark, unsure of how to pray together, consider using these Psalms. In crying out, "How long, Lord?" we can honestly grieve our losses and give them to the One who is capable to hold them. We turn our posture toward Him and allow Him to do the rest.

Though Rebekah was blessed with babies, she unfortunately went on to be less than faithful as she demonstrated favoritism and deceitful behavior in helping her son Jacob steal his brother Esau's birthright. Yet God was faithful to His promises. God carried on the Abrahamic covenant blessing through Jacob just as He said He would. Jacob would take a journey to find a godly wife to secure the family line and blessing, just like the one that was done for his father. God was weaving a story of redemption that led to Jesus, our Messiah.

Rachel

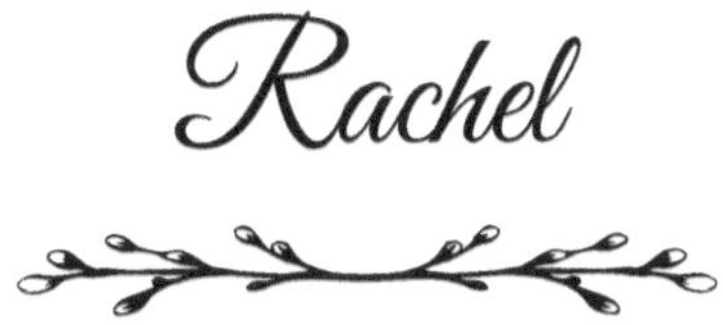

*R*achel seemed to have it all. She was beautiful and married to a man who would carry the lineage of Israel. But in an unjust turn of events, she had to share him with her sister. Jacob, her husband, had been duped by her father into marrying her sister Leah first. In order to marry her as well, he had to work fourteen years for her father. Jacob deeply loved Rachel and only really wanted to be with her. But envy crept in when Leah started pushing out babies left and right, threatening Rachel's role as his favored wife. Leah had four baby boys before the pangs of jealousy were intolerable. Rachel lashed out, "'Give me children or I'll die!'" (Genesis 30:1 NIV).

"I wish I could do it for you; it's easy for me," a coworker said from across the picnic table at a going away party. Upon hearing those words, I froze, even though I'd heard some version of this at least a hundred times before, all with different intonations and intentions. Some altruistic, others pitying, and some offering shame up on a silver platter. In this instance, I know she meant well, but my hurt got the better of me.

"Do you know what it's like?" I asked.

She looked at me expectantly.

Silence.

"It's like we both are applying for a job," I told her. "I get out my best business suit, the one with a matching skirt. I make sure it's ironed—no, better—*dry cleaned.* My best heels. The no-funny-business ones. My resume is pristine, because I have poured over it numerous times. I am fit for the job, a shoo-in. I check all the boxes. I'm an excellent candidate. I even know the owner of the company. There is no good reason for them not to hire me. Then you go to the interview in a bathing suit, with no resume. You have no clue what the company is about. You walked by and they had open interviews, and you thought, 'Well, hey, why not try?' And somehow—you get the job. Not me. And you and everyone else keeps getting the job."

I picked up my plate and left the party.

Friends, if you or someone you love has been on this journey for any length of time, it's likely that you (or they) have suffered under the weight of jealousy or comparison. Despite my best efforts, I found it difficult to avoid taking it personally every time someone announced they were pregnant. Unconsciously, I felt God was limiting His goodness to me and giving it to everyone else. I was triggered often as pregnant bellies swelled everywhere—church, Bible study, the grocery store. Invitations to baby showers, gender reveals, and baby announcements filled my mailbox. It was never-ending, just a matter of time before the next one came. Envy lurked at every corner. My thoughts easily spiraled into despair. The Bible tells us, "Envy rots the bones" (Proverbs 14:30 NIV), and "...Where jealousy and selfish ambition exist, there will be disorder" (James 3:16 ESV). I felt disordered when I fixated on what I didn't have. Jealousy was the rot that ate me alive from the inside out.

And sometimes the jealousy wasn't just about a baby in someone else's arms; it was envy of the steady faith of those who shared my story. As I moved from barren in body to barren in faith, I became convinced the test God had given me was more than I could handle. Unlike me, a friend of mine endured several miscarriages and seemed to just float right along, unbothered, at peace to have Jesus take the wheel. And I couldn't help but say, "God, I'm not sure You picked the right one for this. I'm too emotional. I must be such a disappointment to You." I felt as though I was drowning in fear and doubts in contrast to my friend, who appeared to skip right through the same valley we both were in.

Looking back years later, I see things a little differently. I'd felt defeated at the time, because I only saw pieces, not the full picture. In all honesty, we have no idea if this journey is easier on the person we compare ourselves to. Because it's never the same exact journey. They may have started with a deeper faith, but maybe that's because they had already experienced deeper valleys.

The Bible gives us an example of comparison with Peter when he measured himself against John (John 21). Both he and John were Jesus's disciples and played key roles in the growth of the church. Jesus had just restored Peter for denying Him three times. He moved on to commission Peter to shepherd His people, but Peter deflected the whole conversation, distracted by John. John was another apostle who was self-described as "the one Jesus loved." Peter probably thought, "John has it together. He leaned on You, he's the one You love, and he didn't deny You like I did. What are the plans for him?" The work Jesus was calling him to in that moment was critical to the greater kingdom, and he almost missed it because of comparison.

In John 21:22 Jesus said that we must follow Him. It's as simple as that. Peter would later be the rock to build the church. He had his own calling to fulfill.

Friend, here's what I do know. Jesus knows my heart way better than I ever will. He knew the exact timing when my heart would be able to respond to the crushing, to the weight of grief, to the calling that He gave me. Because, yes, this journey is a calling. If He gave me this transforming catalyst at a different time, when my faith was stronger, my family situation was different, or when I had more financial stability, I wouldn't be here today sharing my story with you. Our Father gives us each a road to travel that is tailored just for us. He is the One who knows what we need, when we need it, and how it will transform us. Because this is a transforming journey, friend. You will either transform to His likeness or fall to doubt, jealousy, and bitterness. You choose. He may have given someone else this trial when her faith was stronger. But maybe I was the one who needed greater transformation, at just the right time, and with the right catalyst resulting in the greater glorification of His work in me.

Let's return to Rachel and Leah. Like any sad story, there are always two sides. While the circumstances were truly unfair for Rachel, Leah was in a valley of her own, enduring a loveless relationship with her husband. He didn't love her, but still slept with her. God saw that she was not loved and He blessed her in that season of sadness, making her fruitful. We get hints of her emotional state in her declarations after each child was born. Each child's name reflected longing, misery, and rejection. Rachel coveted Leah's fruitfulness and lashed out at her husband, demanding that he give her children, or she would die. Her infertility had consumed her to the point that death seemed better than a life without children.

Have you felt at moments that you might die? That your heart was being ripped from your chest? Miscarriages, adoption losses, and negative pregnancy tests may feel like the death of your soul. The understanding and empathy for infertility and pregnancy loss sometimes feels lacking. There are so many unknowns, and the conversation always seems to be behind closed doors, in whispered voices. Many agree that it should be better acknowledged, respected, and understood in medical and emotional spheres. While I personally wasn't experiencing my own death, my heart felt like it was in failure, as though part of me was dying each day. Maybe if it was seen as a complex illness, there would be better research with a clear treatment plan. Maybe friends and family would better understand it and there wouldn't be an uncomfortable silence when our "problem" was brought up. There wouldn't be the bitter taste of shame.

We can see through Rachel how inability to conceive can overtake your whole being to the point of death. It consumed me, too. Once I believed that God didn't want good things for me, it was easy to slide into a thought pattern where I was the one controlling my own outcomes, timed lovemaking encounters, carefully budgeted finances, medications and procedures, keto-genic diets, and scheduled blood draws. These in themselves are not a bad thing as they are necessary in baby making for those who are challenged. The problem was I believed I was in control of my destiny. Not God. This is the tightrope we all walk.

So, will we give it to the Lord, or tightly grip our desire for a baby in our own clenched fists? These desires are given by Him, but when we place our own will above His, they are an idol. How easily that coin flips without us even being aware of it. Increasing negative thoughts, isolation, dwindling prayer and Bible time, and impatience with those around me were some of the alarms going off that I put on snooze. I was consumed to the point of death, because if it wasn't God's will for me to have a baby in my timing, I surely would rather die. Just like Rachel.

There is a caution emerging here for us: Even something as pure as the God-given desire for a child can replace the hope we have in God himself. It can take the throne in our hearts. There is a tenuous balance to be maintained in the pursuit of mother-hood. We must always be seeking the Lord in our pursuit. Some-times the thing we seek wholeheartedly consumes our mind, thoughts, actions—our lives. I wobbled back and forth between God-driven and Heather-driven actions on a daily, often minute-to-minute, basis. It felt like a tug-of-war rope held to the tightest tension, straining back and forth. Me holding the control—injecting the drugs, checking the lists, becoming frustrated with the fertility nurses who were not clear with their instructions, becoming impatient with erratic ovulatory schedules—versus God, who knew the outcome of my striving.

So, what was Jacob's response to Rachel's claims that she would die if she didn't get pregnant? He said, "'Am I in the place of God, who has kept you from having children?'"(Genesis 30:2

NIV). Look at the two things happening here. Jacob rightly defined his role in this debacle, which was that he was under the rule and timing of the Lord. And look what other truth bomb he dropped: God has kept you from having children.

Friends, this is a large pill to swallow. Jacob identified God's knowledge of and authority in the conflict that had engulfed Rachel's and his life. Maybe he accepted it; maybe he was angry about it. But there's a cutting point of truth in his words. *Would God allow this to happen to me? Is it God who kept me from having children? What about sin and its effect in a fallen world? What role do these play in my deep struggle?*

A pastor's wife once said to me, "Heather, God is in charge of wombs. He chooses when they open and when they are closed." I have rolled this idea over and over in my mind like a washing machine on sanitary cycle.

Does He know? Yes.

Did He always know this would happen to me? Yes.

Did He allow it? Yes.

Is this world broken? Most definitely.

And can I let go of trust and allow myself to be led by Him even if it doesn't end the way I want? This is true submission. This is trust. This is the point where we choose to stay, or we choose to leave.

The biggest mistake I made in my wrestling was believing the lies the enemy told me about God. I could grasp that God had allowed this hardship, but I couldn't understand why He wouldn't fix it even though He could. Then, the poison leaked in: I started to believe He didn't care about what was happening to me. That He stood over there aloof and apathetic. He watched me in my pain, but didn't do anything about it. I believed what grieved me didn't grieve Him, which couldn't be farther from the truth. I moved away in my own pain, in my own strength, and in my own bitterness. And instead of transforming, I started pointing a finger. Instead of leaning in, I became consumed with my lack. I grew more and more distant from Him as I listened to the enemy about who He was and made my own version of this "father" built on the lies that were whispered in my ear.

Like Rachel, I wrestled with putting words around what God was doing and where He was when things got difficult. One phrase that I never could wrap my mind around was, "Heather, God is telling you *no*." While I do think there's some evidence behind God saying no, I have long struggled with this narrative. What does it mean? And why do we say it to each other? I don't think it's quite so simple, friends. These are the words our finite minds understand, but tragic events and their reasoning do not always align with human understanding. That's because these things are only known to the Creator of the Universe. Thank goodness, right? If I could fully wrap my mind around an Incarnate, All-powerful, Infinite God, what does that say about who I believe Him to be?

When I was in my season of losses, I was studying the story of King David and the death of his illegitimate child from 2 Samuel 12:13–24 with my local women's Bible group. David fervently prayed for that child to live, and even so, the child ultimately died. The story followed David as he eventually moved from grief-ridden to at peace with what the Lord decided. Two women in our group shared their stories of when their husbands died years before. They revealed how they pleaded with the Lord, but ultimately, it was in the Lord's will to take them to heaven. This moved the conversation to the idea that God said no to their prayers. I don't know why she thought this was okay, but in front of everyone, our leader turned to me and asked me if I would be willing to share about how the Lord had said no to me with my very recent miscarriage.

My face burned with shame and tears pricked the corners of my eyes. Freshly grieving, I was in no position to share in an open forum like this. Despite my request to keep my miscarriage confidential, word of it quickly spread to others in the group, many of whom barely knew my name, never mind my heart.

I stammered a response saying something about trusting in the Lord and His perfect timing. On top of feeling exposed, I felt like a hypocrite—privately, I was painfully wrestling daily with the Lord's goodness (or lack thereof). I struggled to find a desire to talk to a God who was supposedly good but had allowed my baby, one He created naturally in my womb, to die. I led groups with a mask plastered on, pointing women to God, while inside I could hardly face Him. I asked God over and over again, *Why?*

I will say it again: If you are going through something like this, be sure to have a group of people you can trust. This is beyond crucial. Friend, you may feel like you must walk this journey alone, but this is far too much to bear. Many have gone before you and know the way. I'll be honest with you; my pool was and continues to be small. What you have been through, perhaps only few have experienced. Yet, there are some who have not experienced infertility or loss but are willing to climb into those deep waters with you. What a great gift these wonderful people were and continue to be in my life. Despite how much you want to hide and avoid your problem, God created us for each other. This path was never to be walked alone.

To process this "God told you no" moment, I invited a few dear friends from my small group to dinner and shared what had happened. They listened carefully and supportively. When I finished my story, they pushed their chairs back, stunned. They encouraged me to press on and to forgive. They prayed with me. I knew they loved me, and that's what I needed.

I sought counsel with another close friend who I am convinced has a direct line to Jesus. Her sweet young daughter died due to complications of cancer several years earlier. After consoling me, she reminded me that our minds are finite. We do not understand what the Lord understands. We do not see what the Lord sees. We cannot even begin to comprehend His full plan. She was deeply saddened at the idea of someone saying to her that the Lord said no to her prayers when her daughter died. Instead, she looked back at that time as a season when she clung to the Lord. Where her faith was put to fire, and her eyes were fixed on Jesus. She said she would never simplify the shock of that pain as a yes or a no from the Lord. And nor, friends, should we.

What you are going through—not being able to have a baby, losing a baby, not being chosen as an adoptive parent—these may be the darkest times of your life. It does not equate to the Lord saying no to you or me, far from it. It's about saying yes to God in spite of the circumstances. Yes—to His will, His way, His timing. When I choose to say yes to trusting that His plan is better, I choose to believe He holds my breaking heart in His hand, being confident that this journey breaks His heart too. Even when I can't begin to comprehend this situation, He is trustworthy.

For those who are in a supportive role, you may find yourself in a place of not knowing what to say to your struggling loved one and wanting to avoid a situation like I went through. This is a normal response and, quite frankly, it's better to tell your person you don't know what to say rather than giving advice. So often, when we see our loved one in pain, we want to provide a quick fix for their situation, which often causes more hurt. As Esther Fleece notes in her book, *No More Faking Fine*, "We don't always know the reason for another's suffering, and we certainly aren't privy to God's plans or timing to bring them through it. Therefore, it's better to sit with a lamenting person rather than attempting to fix him or her. None of us needs correction to our theology when we are in the depths of our pain. We must resist the urge to offer quick-fix solutions, however well-intentioned" (Fleece, 2017, 184).

Rachel and Leah continued to be rivals, and both women suffered under tremendous stress due to their life circumstances. Rachel was unable to bear children, and Leah responded by leveraging her fertility to get noticed by Jacob, which further exploited her sister's childlessness. Rachel changed her strategy by giving her servant Bilhah to Jacob to start her family line. Rachel must not have gotten the memo from her husband's grandmother, Sarah, that this type of family building only comes with more trouble.

Bilhah had two sons and we see how Rachel felt about herself in the meaning behind their names: "God has vindicated me" and "I won in the struggle against my sister." She felt vindicated from the great weight of shame she felt in her inability to bear a child. Once that was lifted, she viewed family building as a competition between her and her sister. Leah's womb eventually closed as well, so she, too, offered her maidservant to Jacob to produce more children. Leah's servant had two more sons for her. Without a doubt, this was an incredibly complicated family tree with lots of unique branches, but it wasn't beyond God's plan.

Now since both women suffered from closed wombs, they sought the fertility aid of that time—mandrakes. Mandrakes were a plant known to boost fertility. Leah's son happened to find them in the fields and Rachel asked for some. She presented Leah with an offer of a night with their husband in exchange for the mandrakes. Leah accepted the deal, explaining to their husband he must sleep with her because she had hired him. The level of dysfunction is disheartening. All parties had sacrificed their integrity in a contest of growing their family the biggest.

Of note is my personal conviction that seeking modern-day science and fertility to aid in conception is not morally wrong. Many may disagree with me, and that's fine. It breaks my heart to see couples weighed down by shame over their fertility choices. My husband and I agonized over the decision to use fertility aids. The idea of intervening at each step of the conception process made me wonder if we weren't letting God be God. If this was His will, would it not just happen on its own? Wouldn't that be a better story to behold? We met with our pastor and his wife to get some biblical insight and support on this difficult decision. I'll never forget the words that my pastor's wife said: "The Lord is always in the room. The Lord is there in that lab when the critical decision for life is made or not made, when those tiny embryo cells develop or remain stagnant." The Lord is there when that embryo is placed in my broken womb and decides to attach or falls away. He is there. He knows. He sees. He allows.

Being a medical provider, I have seen evidence that science and medical knowledge can be God-given and God-inspired. There are ways to engage in reproductive technology while still protecting the integrity of an unborn life. My own reproductive physician, a Christ follower, held my hand and prayed over our very tiny baby after an embryo transfer. The Lord was in that place without question.

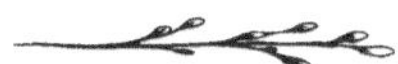

God listened to Leah and she got pregnant after that barter, having another son, and then later a daughter. God continued to bless her by opening her womb. In His goodness, God, too, remembered Rachel. Even in her missteps, God heard her crying heart and was merciful.

What about this business of remembering? Does that mean He forgot her before? No. This same language was used with Noah and the flood (Genesis 8:1). When the Bible says, "God remembered," we are not to understand this as though God forgot something. Rather, we should see God is preparing to deliver on His promise and finish what He started. God remembering is God preparing to act and bring His promise to life (Hayes, 2022). Even more important, God remembering confirmed He would follow through on His covenant promises with His people.

Rachel bore a son, whom she named Joseph, which means "may the Lord add to me another son" (Genesis 30:24 NIV). She said, "'God has taken away my disgrace'" (Genesis 30:23 NIV). She recognized that God had the power to open her womb, and that He heard her prayers. Several years later, Rachel went on to have another son, Benjamin, but she tragically died during that birth. The very thing that caused her hardship and consumed her ended up taking her life.

Ultimately, God was sovereign in Rachel's infertility and the source of blessing that she competed for. God was the one who opened and closed wombs. His plan superseded the plans formulated by Rachel and Leah. Their children would be a part of His covenant with Abraham as each child would represent a future tribe of Israel that would make up the great nation. The promised lineage that extended to Jesus would come from this family tree, which was rooted in barrenness.

Manoah's Wife (Sampson's Mother)

Judges 13

Our next story is one that may be unknown, even to those who are familiar with the Bible. Manoah was more commonly known as Sampson's father. He was a man of Zorah of the tribe of Dan. Though God had given the land of Zorah to the Danites, they struggled to completely possess it from their enemies, the Philistines. Their inability to inhabit the land was attributed to lack of faith (Judges 18:1–31). Manoah was married to an incredibly faithful but infertile woman, referred to only as "Manoah's wife." We do not get the privilege of knowing her name. Judges 13 describes her as "childless and unable to give birth" (Judges 13:3).

One day, an angel of the Lord appeared to her. God has a way of showing up with news, doesn't He? There are four women in the Bible who were told by an angel or Christophany that they would bear a child. Sarah, Manoah's wife, Elizabeth, and Mary. Three out of the four were barren women.

The angel told Manoah's wife she was barren and childless but said she would become pregnant and give birth to a son. When the angel shared the news, he used the word *behold*, not once, but twice (Judges 13:3 NASB). "Behold" means to observe something particularly remarkable. He also had to tell her twice that she would have a son.

I'm thinking of a few things right now. One, we know that it would be quite remarkable (Behold!) for her to be able to produce a baby. The Bible was painfully clear that she was unable to conceive. Two, it was so remarkable she had to be told twice. I'm sure she was jumping up and down for joy with great hopes that her dreams of a child were finally going to come true. Then, the angel gave her the tough news: There would be a cost to this pregnancy. Her son would be dedicated to the Lord from birth which came with some heavy responsibilities.

He would be under her care only for a short while and he, too, would have to follow Nazarite law—no haircuts for him. More importantly, he would help deliver the Israelites from the Philistines. This was of utmost importance as Israel had been in the hands of the Philistines for forty years. The Israelites were desperate for rescue, and Sampson would be the one to get the ball rolling. They needed a rescuer, a redeemer. Does this story sound at all familiar? I love how the Bible is always pointing to Jesus. Jesus was the only one, our Rescuer and Redeemer, who could end the exile of sin when He came to the world years later.

After the angel left, Manoah's wife went to her husband and said, "An awesome man of God, who looked like an angel, came and told me I'm going to have a baby," but her explanation didn't satisfy bewildered Manoah. He desired to hear it for himself. So, he prayed and God sent the angel back for another one-on-one encounter. With his wife. It's interesting that God saw fit to share these important announcements in secret, without Manoah. In fact, it's quite shocking in a time when women were not seen as respected members of society. This special message was bestowed on a woman, not once, but twice! Behold! When the angel appeared to the woman again, she knew she'd better get her husband.

Upon finding the angel, Manoah started questioning him. "What will happen to this child? What will his vocation be?" He had all the questions about the future.

I can't help but think that we were a bit like Manoah. There have been so many instances where I just couldn't logically figure out how the details were going to work out in God's plan. I asked and sometimes demanded that God reveal the future.

Would this baby make it? Should we do genetic testing? What would we do if that testing came back with poor results? What if this baby was born with a congenital defect? We peppered God and our doctors with our questions. We didn't have all of the answers, and I wonder if it was because God wanted us to step into unwavering faith like Manoah's wife.

The angel replied to Manoah that he had given clear directions to his wife. But Manoah tried to stall this heavenly being, so he asked him to stay for dinner. (Important note: celestial beings can't consume meals.)

The angel responded with a different idea. "Give an offering to the Lord instead." Manoah wasn't convinced this was an angel so he pressed the angel to identify himself by name. The angel responded that his name was "Wonderful." Manoah agreed to the sacrifice and suddenly, the angel performed something spectacular and not of this world.

A flame went up from the altar, and the angel ascended into it. Manoah and his wife fell on their faces needing no further convincing that this being was God. However, Manoah became panicked they would die, having seen the Lord. His wife had some sense and told him death was not possible because if the Lord had desired to kill them, He wouldn't have wasted His time going through this whole prophecy. In due time, Manoah's wife bore a son, and she named him Sampson just as she was instructed and the Spirit of the Lord stirred in him.

Here are a few takeaways I gleaned from this story. The angel addressed Manoah's wife as "infertile" more than once. My first response was, "Yeah, no kidding, buddy. I'm sure she already knew that." But in identifying this, the "angel" distinguished who He was and His all-knowing capabilities. He was not a stranger to her situation. He saw her pain and her need. He *came down for her.* His whole purpose of being there was to let her know her story was about to change. He came to *her*, to the woman, to the wife, which was quite radical in those times. Also surprising, the angel met with her twice (perhaps to the dismay of her husband). God was unwavering with His instruction.

Many biblical scholars agree that the angel was the preincarnate Lord. Isaiah 9:6 (NIV) says, "And he will be called Wonderful Counselor." In Hebrew this was written as "*pele*," which correlates with the divine nature of God and means incomprehensible (Bible Hub, 2026). Once the heavenly being went up in a flame, Manoah knew He was Jesus, the Son of God Himself, who had come down to fix what was broken. Manoah's wife didn't need convincing. She knew in her heart when she had first seen Him and she was ready to act on His directions.

It gives me chills to think about. When have I prayed for something, and God showed up in a very real way? When has God directed me on something, then came back to confirm the same instructions I should have just followed in the first place? Where has God been unwavering in His instruction to me?

Manoah's wife had to live a life that was holy and set apart, following Nazarite law while she was pregnant. She had to avoid wine, fermented drink, and all unclean foods. She had to give things up. She had to surrender many of her own expectations of what her pregnancy would be like. But she was seamlessly obedient and gave up her own comforts for a calling.

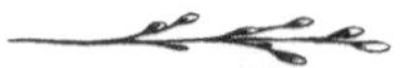

Many of us have adapted to a host of changes in hopes to grow our families. I've eaten McDonald's french fries immediately following an embryo transfer and heart of pineapple during the two-week wait. I've followed various diets and avoided processed and fermented foods. My husband decreased his intake of chicken wings and beer, a sacrifice that grieved him (insert laugh). He had to learn how to give injections into my derrière. We took countless natural supplements in addition to fertility medications. About twenty weeks into my pregnancy with my twins, I was put on bed rest.

I remember being in my busy clinic at the hospital, answering yet another parent phone call, when searing contractions interrupted my words. I set the phone down and put both hands on my tight abdomen. My colleague eyeballed me with a look of worry from across the workroom. Today was not the day. We were short-staffed and I could not afford to take time off because I was saving it for maternity leave. I called Dr. LG's office and spoke to the on-call nurse practitioner, who instructed me to go home or, at the very least, sit as much as I could. She sent a prescription in for medication to help stop the contractions, but it only made me dizzy and sick. I ended up going home, prompting my worried mom to bring over a tub of baby clothes passed on to me from her friend. We oohed and ahhed over each cute onesie, and she laid them over my belly, encouraging the two babies wrestling inside to calm down and stay put.

A week later, at my next appointment, Dr. LG looked me directly in the eye and said, "No more work."

"No more work?" I repeated, glancing over to my husband, who avoided eye contact and shifted in his seat. He knew I wouldn't be happy about this abrupt change. I'd expected to continue work until my third trimester. I was in the middle of launching a pilot clinic, and I could not imagine leaving my patients for an extended period of time. I did not have enough paid time off to cover an extended leave. We had not decorated the nursery or washed even one onesie.

The doctor let me talk myself in circles for several minutes before he said, "You get to do this one time … make the right choice." The very thing I had wanted so badly and had miraculously achieved was coming at an even greater cost. I had to pause my productivity because my body demanded more protection. And in protecting, I had to pause the rest of the only identity I'd known, my career.

Initially, I struggled to let go of my work, busying myself with spreadsheets and data collection that could be done while lying flat. But as time went on, my body and the two babies inside were the ones that convinced me change was inevitable. I realized the critical need for a reset before entering into motherhood, releasing my grip on my career to make room for the greater role ahead of me.

Manoah's wife, on the other hand, seemed to have no issues sliding into the sacrifice of motherhood. She was a woman of unwavering faith and obedience. She did not need that second appearance from the angel for reassurance as her husband did. She knew she was deeply loved by Our Heavenly Father, who came down to earth for her. She knew and instantly believed in her calling. Her tribe and husband may have struggled to trust God fully, but her own faith was steadfast. She willingly prepared to take all responsibilities necessary to be Sampson's mother, no matter the sacrifice.

God saw her obedience and blessed her to be a witness to something truly unexpected and miraculous. As if having a baby was not miraculous enough, she got a teaser of what Jesus's ascension would look like as the angel went up in flames in front of her eyes. Our Deliverer came to save back then and soon will come to save again.

Ruth

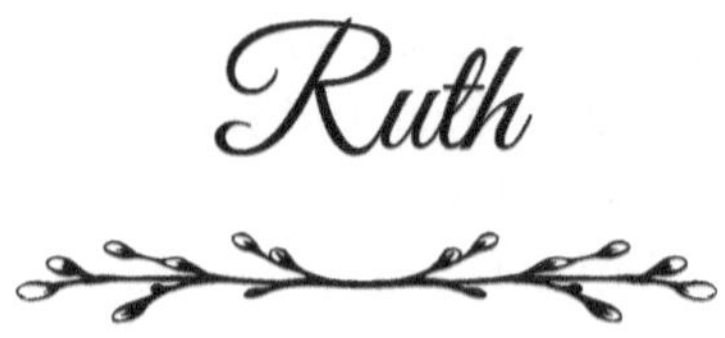

Ruth 1–4

Ruth is another character in the Bible who is not primarily known for infertility, but if we look closely at her story there are clues to show she likely was. Ruth endured the loss of her husband and left everything to live in a foreign land with her bitter mother-in-law. Her story embodies bravery, loyalty, and God's faithful provision. She is known by today's believers as part of the grafting-in of the Gentiles. She is the unexpected character in Jesus's lineage. She's an outsider, a Gentile, a Moabitess.

The Bible tells us Ruth's in-laws and husband were Ephrathites, or residents of Bethlehem. Prophetic Scriptures of Micah record this region as the area where Jesus would come from. The Hebrew word *ephrath* means "fruitful." Fruitful, however, would not describe Ruth and her first husband, Mahlon.

Ruth and Mahlon met when the family moved to Moab due to a famine in Bethlehem. It was surprising that Mahlon took a liking to her, since intermarrying with foreign people was discouraged for Israelites. Moabites were particularly hated by Israel because this people emerged from the incestuous relationship between Lot and his daughter (Genesis 19:36). Israelites were instructed to avoid peace and friendship with Moabites. And yet, Mahlon's family chose to settle there and allowed both boys to marry Moabite women. Naomi, their mother, would have been the one to give the marriage blessing because their father, Elimelek, died soon after they moved. They were married for ten years when both Mahlon and his brother abruptly died. The Bible does not tell us why or how they died. The clue may be in the meaning behind their names: "sickly" and "frail." Neither Ruth nor her Moabite sister-in-law, Orpah, had any children in the ten years they were married. In those days, it would be rare for a couple to have no children after ten years of marriage unless there was a problem.

Naomi, Ruth's mother-in-law, had lost her husband, and now both of her sons. She said she believed the hand of God was against her. She made plans to move back to Bethlehem because she had heard God had relieved His people from the famine. She told Ruth and Orpah to return to their homes and gods to ease their grief, with hopes they would remarry. Initially they protested, but Naomi insisted it was best for everyone. She would not likely remarry, and even if she did, she would not be able to quickly produce sons for them to marry.

Naomi was trying to be merciful to the women as it would have been difficult for a Moabitess to fit into Israelite culture. Naomi may have even realized the critical error her family had made moving to Moab, now after experiencing death in all her immediate family members and seeing God had provided relief from famine in Israel. Orpah agreed to return to her people and gods. Ruth, however, refused to go back and was so determined to stay that Naomi gave up convincing her.

Mahlon's faith may not have been strong enough to turn Ruth to God while he was alive, but it was through his death that Ruth fully received the God of Israel as her Lord. Ruth proclaimed the verses we all know so well. "Where you go, I will go, [...] Your people will be my people and your God my God. (Ruth 1:16–17 NIV).

They carried on and arrived in Bethlehem, and the whole town stirred. Maybe because Naomi arrived with an enemy, or perhaps it was her bitter disposition because her friends said, "Can this be Naomi?"

> "Don't call me Naomi," she told them. "Call me Mara, because the Almighty has made my life very bitter. I

went away full, but the LORD has brought me back empty. Why call me Naomi? The LORD has afflicted me; the Almighty has brought misfortune upon me."

Ruth 1:20–21 NIV

I wonder if Ruth understood how very vulnerable they were. They had no man in sight to defend them and technically no secured land because Naomi was a widow. Without Ruth, Naomi would have been left defenseless and alone, blinded by grief and bitterness, a widow. And yet, Ruth clung to the very hard-to-love Naomi. This was sacrifice. It would have made a hundred times more sense for her to leave. She would have avoided judgment. She would have easily found a new husband with the same cultural and faith background in her hometown. Yet something—or rather, Someone—pointed Ruth's heart to Naomi, and Ruth chose to be all-in.

Contrary to Ruth, Naomi's heart was in a place of famine. She renamed herself bitter. She didn't understand how she fled her home with a full family, only to return with no family. The homeland she left due to famine was now flourishing, and she was the one spiritually and physically starving.

Unknowingly, the women settled near a man related to Naomi's late husband. God is the God of details here. He directed Ruth and Naomi to this place that had been there all along to ensure they were provided for. Ruth was able to glean the fields— that is, collect food left behind by harvesters. She worked alone, making her increasingly vulnerable. Boaz, the field's owner, inquired about Ruth when he saw her picking. When he was told she was Naomi's daughter-in-law, he asked her to stay in his fields to ensure her protection. He shared a meal with her, encouraging her to eat as much as she wanted. She asked why he was being so kind to her, and he said her reputation for caring for her mother-in-law proceeded her. He increased her gleaning abilities by allowing her to move alongside the harvesters.

Naomi was stunned by this farmer's generosity, and after a quick round of Dutch bingo, she discovered Boaz was their family's guardian kinsman redeemer. A kinsman redeemer is a close male relative who serves as a helper to a family whose head of home had died. Their duties included buying a family member out of slavery, avenging murder, buying back forfeited land, and safeguarding persons, property, and inheritance that belonged to the family. He would be their rescuer. God exceedingly provided for Ruth and Naomi, not just in food but by precisely placing them next to the family protection they desperately needed.

At the beginning of our journey, after several months without answers, our reproductive endocrinologists recommended that we move to higher-level treatment: in vitro fertilization. A treatment that involves extensive testing, manipulation, procedures, and you guessed it, *cost*. The doctors still had no idea why I couldn't get pregnant. We were out of money, exhausted in emotion and body, and feeling hopeless. We thought it best to take some time to pray, rethink, and repurpose. The question, "have you considered adoption?" kept finding its way into our conversations. I think often many of us who are on this journey are advised to consider adoption without much thought. Though the suggestion may come with good intent, I would implore anyone to do their research before offering this idea.

Brent had been listening to a sermon series on adoption and was feeling led to pray about it. It wasn't that we hadn't entertained the idea of adoption before. We had attended adoption information sessions for both local and international adoption. We had a connection with the country of Haiti having done prior mission work there. However, we kept running into roadblocks. The Hague Adoption Convention, which was the authority on adoption protocols for international countries, had closed Haiti for adoption which shut that door.

We quickly found adopting a child often required a vetting higher than any other life decision. The cost started at $20,000 and only went up from there. The price tag is even higher today. There are legal ramifications, medical assessments, background checks, invasive home studies, and expectations which well exceed the standard checklist of biological parenthood. While pursuing adoption, we found our marriage license had a clerical error which would prevent us from proceeding forward. I spent hours at the State of Michigan court being passed from person to person to rectify this error.

We explored the great responsibilities associated with taking on the role as adoptive parents. We met with a lawyer who grilled us on personal matters, from our choice of pets to whether we had ever used hard drugs which would immediately take us out of the running as adoptive parents. We considered how to honor an adoptive child's cultural or racial backgrounds and if they would acclimate into our community. We were posed with the possibility of adopting a child who had been abused, drug-exposed, or had special needs. We contemplated changing our lives by moving and leaving our jobs to accommodate the needs of our potential child.

While I have not personally experienced an adoption loss or disrupted adoption, I've heard many heart-wrenching stories of couples experiencing the unknowns and whiplash related to failed placements or disrupted adoption. These heartaches echo the loss we all endure. Barrenness is not just a condition of the body, it's a condition of the heart. Adoption should not be lightly suggested. As much as it hurt to hear, the counselor was right to say we needed to be at peace with our infertility before pursuing adoption. This process was not for the weak of heart, and our hearts were bleeding.

We were able to find an agency that was supportive of us pursuing adoption while considering fertility treatments. We started filling out the paperwork. As with any attempt at procuring a baby—by science or otherwise—a check needed to be written. We had carefully filled out the paperwork and had a deposit check to deliver to the agency the next day. That evening, in the middle of the night, I lost consciousness from abdominal pain when getting up to go to the bathroom.

Pain had been a common symptom for me and something I paid little attention to as I figured this might be expected when one takes a pharmacy worth of drugs to reverse infertility. In fact, in my younger days, I was often found asleep on the stairs after passing out from pain during a menstrual cycle. In college, I split my chin open after passing out in the shower. I was told many women in my family had "hard" periods and several had hysterectomies at young ages, so I just assumed it must be "normal" to have this type of pain. This wasn't normal. And perhaps the answers we were looking for were right in front of me all along.

At that moment, everything was put on hold, including our adoption papers. I was seen urgently by a surgeon who was confident there was a pathologic cause for both our infertility and my pain. Endometriosis. My surgery showed widespread aggressive disease throughout my uterus, bladder, and intestine—stage four—the most severe type. Our surgeon had done his best to remove it, but his recommendation was to use hormone suppression to try to calm the inflammation inside my body. And our best bet at effective hormone suppression was pregnancy.

I felt like I would never get off this awful merry-go-round. I was at a complete loss. I was bitter. On a journey in search of a full family, I was given a new chronic disease and was right back to the barren place I started. Like Naomi, I started winding my identity around bitterness. I felt as though God's hand was against me. I was beyond frustrated. Nothing was working and more things kept going wrong. I didn't know why He would allow this to happen and why there was no solution. No peace. Only heartache.

We were broke and had no idea how we would fund a round of IVF. IVF was not covered by our insurance and costs ballooned well into $30,000 per round. We started strategizing on how to quickly save money. We sold furniture, household items, and things we no longer needed. We made a spreadsheet to keep track of the dollars that we were able to collect. We ate cheap noodles. We cut our cable and all extra subscriptions. We applied for jobs in states that mandated fertility insurance coverage. We considered working for Starbucks (one of the first companies that offered insurance covering the cost of fertility treatments). We worried. We spent time on our knees.

Until one day, when Brent brought home a document that contained his health benefits, including a fund he had (unknowingly) been putting money into since the day he started his job. Today you and I would know this as a Health Savings Account. It contained several thousand dollars eligible to be used for fertility treatments. We looked at each other stunned. We checked and double-checked that the balance was correct. We called twice to ensure the funds were eligible to be used for reproductive therapy. An undiscovered cache of provision was there all along that we could glean. God had gone ahead of us, scattering what we had needed before knew we would need it, just as He had in the field for Ruth. Provision. Abundant provision. God is the God of details. We were able to move forward to treatment immediately.

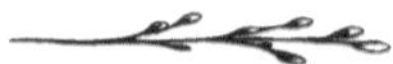

Ruth continued gleaning until harvest season ended, while Naomi took on the role as matchmaker. Ruth needed a husband for her future security. So Naomi directed Ruth to put on her best outfit, spray herself with perfume, and go to the threshing floor where Boaz was winnowing barley. She was to lay down at his feet and wait for him to tell her what to do.

Following winnowing season, there was a celebration for farmers and their workers. They would eat and drink together, happy the hard labor was over. It was a bit of a scandal for Naomi to direct Ruth to lay at Boaz's feet after a night of partying, but Boaz had already shown himself as a man of integrity in all the ways he took care of Ruth. You might ask why was this man sleeping on the floor in his barn? In those times of political instability, thievery was extremely common. It was a normal practice for field owners to sleep with their harvested crops to protect against attacks.

Lying at Boaz's feet on the threshing floor was an act of submission, and Ruth took it a bit further by basically proposing to Boaz. She asked him to spread his garment over her. Spreading a skirt over a widow was a way of claiming a wife. This is still practiced today in Jewish weddings, when the man throws the end of his talith (shawl) over his new wife to signify she is under his protection (Guzik, 2025).

It was Ruth's right as Mahlon's widow to demand a kinsman redeemer's safeguarding over her family, property, and inheritance. But she laid down her own rights by laying humbly at his feet. In lying at his feet, she said, "I respect you, and I trust you to make the right decision for me."

Boaz accepted Ruth's proposal and put Ruth under his protection with blessings. As kinsman redeemer, he could have forced his rights on her. He could have taken advantage of her and her family's land, but he didn't. He was a gentleman. Still there was one more barrier to overcome; there was a closer kinsman redeemer than Boaz. This man already had a wife and family who could be negatively impacted by their union. Commentaries state that marrying Ruth would likely result in additional children, who would increase the competition for the combined estate with his existing sons.

The next morning Ruth left and Boaz went to settle things with the closer kinsman redeemer. That man deferred to Boaz to redeem Ruth's family with all the elders present to witness the transaction. The elders blessed Boaz and Ruth, asking God to make Ruth like Rachel and Leah. *Rachel and Leah.* You heard it right. While they eventually produced a large family tree, both suffered from infertility. Now they were recognized as the foundation for the line of Israel. A blessing of fertility rooted in a barren history.

After marrying Boaz, the Lord enabled Ruth to conceive (because she was prior unable), and she had a son named Obed. Obed, the father of Jesse, who was the father of David, whose lineage traces to Jesus. Ruth, a Moabitess, an assumed enemy of Israel, infertile, grafted into Israelite lineage and directly linked to Jesus.

Naomi's friends surrounded her, praising the Lord, because He did not leave her without a redeemer. They said, "...your daughter-in-law, who loves you and who is better to you than seven sons, has given him birth" (Ruth 4:15 NIV). This was a blessing—in ancient days, seven sons equaled the ideal family. Ruth, an infertile foreign daughter-in-law was more valuable to Naomi than seven coveted sons. Ruth was the best blessing imaginable. They also said, "Naomi has a son" (Ruth 4:17 NIV). Well, actually, a grandson, right? It was through Obed, that the lineage of Israel to Jesus was again restored. Obed was the "son" Naomi needed to prevent her family line from vanishment. She had been restored with a full family once again. She had safety and security restored. No longer would she identify as bitter, but as blessed.

This story is evidence of Joel 2:25 (NIV) in perfect human form. "I will repay you for the years the locusts have eaten." Ruth experienced shame, emptiness, and great loss, and yet her life is a testimony that God does not waste devastation. He is the great Restorer.

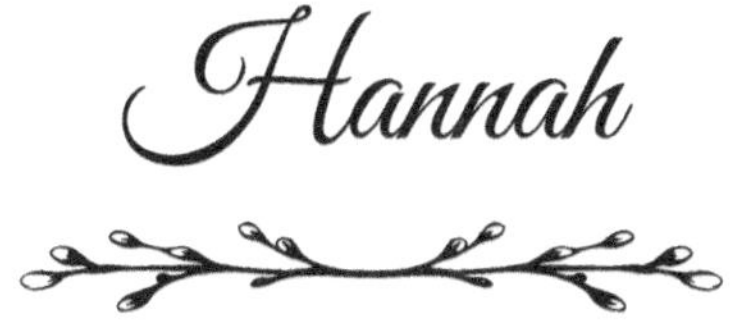Hannah

1 Samuel 1–2:21

There was a certain man from Ramathaim, a Zuphite from the hill country of Ephraim, whose name was Elkanah […] He had two wives; one was called Hannah and the other Peninnah. Peninnah had children, but Hannah had none.

Year after year this man went up from his town to worship and sacrifice to the Lord Almighty at Shiloh, where Hophni and Phinehas, the two sons of Eli, were priests of the Lord. Whenever the day came for Elkanah to sacrifice, he would give portions of the meat to his wife Peninnah and to all her sons and daughters. But to Hannah he gave a double portion because he loved her, and the LORD had closed her womb.

1 Samuel 1:1–5 NIV

*H*annah was adored by her husband, Elkanah. Seems to be a common thread in these biblical women, right? First Rebekah, then Rachel, now Hannah. But shame ruined their annual trip to the house of the Lord. Each year the same thing happened: the family went to temple, offered sacrifice, and shared the sacrificial meal. Elkanah, in charge of divvying it up, always gave Hannah the double portion. Peninnah, the other wife, got jealous, then provoked Hannah.

The prized double portion meal should have gone to the oldest son. Deuteronomy 21:15–17 lays out the law regarding how rights and inheritances should be divided in families. The double portion was meant for the firstborn son, regardless of the father's favor. Yet, Elkanah broke tradition and gave it to Hannah. Did Hannah just look hangry? Did she need more food than the average woman? Maybe he thought feeding her more would help promote fertile hormones? Perhaps he loved her so much because she wanted to give him children but couldn't. It wasn't that he didn't have a firstborn son; Peninnah had produced one for him which probably enraged her more, as her son was denied the blessing that he rightfully deserved. Remember, Peninnah, like Leah, was unloved. Wrong or right, she had her own reasons to act out. Hannah was seen and deeply loved by her husband, but she missed it because her vision was clouded by Peninnah's bullying.

Has this happened to you? Has something provoked the pain you already carry? Life does not stop marching on, even when we are laid out by grief. Over the years, I had experienced my parents' divorce, job loss, the death of a close friend and neighbor, among many other disappointments. It wasn't one person who provoked me. It was life itself, each heartbreak snowballing upon another. I had to learn to cope with long-standing grief piled on by more grief.

After the death of my friend and a recent miscarriage, I told my therapist, "I just want to be done."

She gently pressed me. "Heather, you can't rush dealing with grief. I know you have coped this way before, but now … your body is telling you it's too much."

She was right.

I wanted to be "myself" again. I wanted to push through with denial. I knew I was easily distracted, and I didn't carry my usual level of sincerity. I couldn't be present in conversations. I was exhausted. I didn't have capacity. I wanted to get off the grief merry-go-round. Every ounce of emotional energy was given to keeping the mask on and getting through the day. Though my heart was broken, life moved on. The world kept turning even when mine was falling apart. I still had a job to do, I still had to be a mother, I still needed to show up for the people who needed me. Many whom I interacted with daily did not know my story. Some did, but were uncomfortable talking about it, or were too quick to offer "a fix." I struggled to assume the best of those around me while trying to keep my head above the waves of grief. I found it easier to keep the raw areas closed. My heart could only stand to share so many times, and reliving the grief was draining. I tried my best to just push through, until there was no more pushing that could be done.

> Whenever Hannah went up to the house of the LORD, her rival provoked her till she wept and would not eat. Her husband Elkanah would say to her, "Hannah, why are you weeping? Why don't you eat? Why are you downhearted? Don't I mean more to you than ten sons?"
>
> 1 Samuel 1:7–8 NIV

In her grief, Hannah stopped eating. Ironically, she got the double portion, but she couldn't eat it. Elkanah said to her, "Am I not worth ten sons?" *This man.* He felt the deep weight of her pain. He didn't put pressure on her to produce more sons for him. He desperately wanted to have value in her eyes that were clouded by her own lack. This type of love was rare—extremely rare in that cultural time. Those were times that allowed men to freely divorce their wives if it was determined they were infertile, no questions asked. Elkanah's was extravagant love. Sacrificial love.

Take some time to consider the sacrifices your husband has made for you. I don't know about you, but often I was so lost in my own thoughts, so consumed with what was in front of me, that I didn't see him. Maybe these sacrifices are obvious ones—the medical workup he's done, the thankless job he works to pay for adoption fees, the injections he's helped give, the medications he's picked up, the hugs he's offered when the month passes and there's another negative test. And maybe some not-so-obvious—loyalty to you when others don't understand your story or choices, trust in your decision-making, restraint when your emotions and words are all over the place, a safe embrace to fall into when your dreams are falling apart. He, too, experiences the same heartache.

He may feel rejection just as Elkanah did. "Don't I mean more to you than ten sons?" *Alright, Elkanah, it's not all about you.* But it's clear, he didn't feel seen. Do you know how valuable ten sons were back then? And they meant more to Hannah than they did to him. It's so crucial to stop to see these tender actions. The double portion that was willingly given to you. These actions bond a marriage together in the most difficult of times. I think of the times my husband sat with me in the bathroom waiting for the pregnancy test result, how he carried me up the stairs after my D&C, how he intervened in unheard conversations with assuming relatives. These will be the times you look back on as refining in your relationship. I want to gently encourage you to look for these moments, to acknowledge them, and to be grateful for them.

After they finished eating, something in Hannah told her to go to the house of the Lord. "In her deep anguish Hannah prayed to the LORD, weeping bitterly" (1 Samuel 1:10 NIV).

My mind drifts back to a time most of us keep locked in the recesses of our mind. Those moments when we hit rock bottom racked with grief and absolute outrage. The dark night of the soul when we think, *this couldn't be a God who loves me.* The moments we contemplate walking away.

I was naturally and unexpectedly pregnant, again. This was my second natural unexpected pregnancy. My body was willing to conceive, but unable to carry a baby much beyond the second trimester. I started to feel dread about the possibility of the thing I had wanted the most. My husband had just had elective foot surgery and was hobbling around in a plastic boot. My obstetrician was carefully and aggressively monitoring this pregnancy. I already had many reassuring lab results and had seen two ultrasounds indicating our baby was appropriately growing. We had heard the tiny bleeps of our baby's steady heartbeat.

One afternoon, I sat in my OB's office on my lunch break, waiting over an hour because he was running behind. I shifted on the paper-lined table uncomfortably careful not to unhinge the safety pin holding my pants together. Given I had been pregnant so many times before, my body obligingly showed the signs. I was thirteen weeks pregnant, through the first trimester, when most women breathe a sigh of relief. Yet, I was too guarded to do that.

Dr. LG rushed through the door and ushered me back to the ultrasound room I had been in so many times before. The tech waited for me while he moved on to see another patient. I lay on the bed and turned to look at the ultrasound screen. I held my breath. The fuzzy images cleared to show a tiny unmoving body. The tech jiggled the ultrasound wand a bit and pushed on my abdomen. The little body remained still. We both stared at the screen, willing for it to move. Air left my lungs and tears spilled down my cheeks as she deftly left the room to find the doctor.

I whipped out my phone and texted a coworker, asking her to tell my office manager I had to go home sick. She knew what was up; her own story was very similar to mine. She answered back, "No, it can't be. Please no." My doctor rushed in, grabbed the ultrasound probe, and we saw my unmoving sweet little baby again. I watched as he moved it around carefully, observing each facet of my precious deceased child. I marveled at the definition, hands, feet, a little head and belly. Never to see this side of heaven.

He stated, "The baby is intact with no obvious deformities. It must be chromosomal."

I could no longer look at the screen and softly started to sob.

He held my hand and asked how he could help. His eyes scanned the room. "Where's Brent?"

I mumbled, "Foot surgery yesterday…no time off…he's not here." I was so vulnerable and alone.

He quietly asked what I wanted to do. "We can wait. It should pass on its own," he murmured.

I interrupted him, knowing my history of pregnancy loss ending in a D&C. "Get it out," I told him. "I want it out."

He nodded knowingly and ducked out of the room to make arrangements. I called my husband at work, and he was at a loss for words while machines stamped away in the background. A nurse came in and drew my blood for the surgery to remove my baby the next day. I heard sounds of patients being seen across the hall. Pregnant patients with live babies inside their bellies, newborn babies being seen during post-partum appointments. I couldn't stand to look at my own belly. The four walls closed in on me as they handed me my pre-op paperwork for the next day, and I tripped over myself to get out of the room.

I got to the parking lot and called my sister, asking her to babysit the boys the next day. I choked out the words, telling her I was pregnant. She didn't know; no one did except us. She was dumbfounded but quickly agreed to watch the kids. I numbly drove home. I walked in my house and looked around lost, as if it was the first time I had been there. In my bedroom, I lay in the fetal position, grabbed a pillow, and screamed into it.

And then I got on my knees and cried out to the Lord, "How could you? How could you do this to me? I did not ask for this. I did not pray for this. If You were such a merciful God, You would have not allowed me to get pregnant in the first place. You… are…cruel." My words were incomprehensible by broken sobs. Racked with grief. Crying out to the Lord. Anguished.

Hannah, deeply anguished herself, began bargaining with God. She made a vow offering the up the very gift she pled for. If the Lord would remember her by giving her a child, she would offer him in service. She whispered these words in her heart, her mouth moving as she cried out.

Eli, a priest in the temple, spied these actions and assumed she was drunk. He offended her, telling her to lay off the wine. When she explained she was pouring out her soul, she wasn't drunk, he responded, "Whatever it is that you are asking for, may God grant it to you."

Real meaningful, right? It almost feels flippant. Easy button! May God give it to you. No treatments, no adoption papers, no hemorrhaging financials, no fear of miscarriage. Simple. This would have saved Rachel a whole lot of trouble with those mandrakes. Here's the most important thing, we should not underestimate the power prayer has on our lives. Eli didn't even know what he was asking of God. He just said, whatever your problem is, may God grant what you ask. In that moment, heaven opened up.

Countless people have prayed for me over the years. I had a friend who wore a ring on her finger to remind her to pray for me throughout the day while we were waiting for IVF results. I had sweet sisters in faith lay hands on me and pray for God's direction for fertility treatments. My Reproductive Endocrinologist prayed over me after he performed an embryo transfer.

I have offered intercessory prayers for others. One for a sweet friend, whose dog tragically died while she was out of state undergoing IVF treatments. An early morning prophetic awakening prompted me to pray, and the Lord plainly revealed to me she would hold this child in her arms. I had no choice but to call her immediately and tell her this hopeful news. His name is Samuel. He's five years old today.

People of all types have prayed. I'll be honest. I'm not sure they were all genuine. Only God knew their hearts. Maybe deep inside resided judgment about our choice to use reproductive medicine, a conviction about adoption, discomfort around talking about fertility, or something else that held their hearts back. I heard a pastor on the radio once say his first response after hearing an infertility story was to immediately pray with the couple the moment he found out. To pray with them. Right then and there, because we never know where God is on His timeline. We do not know the moment heaven will open allowing a heart to be transformed, hope restored, supernatural peace poured out, or even a miracle revealed.

Now don't get me wrong, I'm not saying prayer equals a

miracle or a baby. I've offered up many a prayer that went unanswered or was answered by God saying, "Wait." But each prayer shifted my heart a little more toward His. Each prayer brought me into a place of reliance where I could release my control, saying, "God, this situation isn't mine. It was always Yours." Prayer aligns our hearts in the correct position with His, which is crucial for this journey. Know that I intercede for you as I write these words. Don't give up praying.

Eli's prayer brought Hannah to a place of hope. Her face was no longer downcast; she ate. She went to worship the next morning. Read it again. *She went to worship.* Do you feel as though you are walking in the dark right now? Are you desperately looking for relief that can't be found? Do you feel the anguish that she did?

What would it look like to go to a place of worship? Maybe that's in a church pew, or maybe it's a walk on the beach, or another place that brings peace. Your special place or that spot where God feels near. For me, worship was found in His creation on hikes. In other seasons, it was found in a hammock in a friend's Chicago backyard. It was a place where I found safety and solace. A place I could pour out my soul and feel no shame or anxiety. Is there a place that feels this way for you? Be sure to find this rest for your soul.

The Lord remembered Hannah. Here's that word again. It doesn't mean He forgot her. As we discussed with Rachel, *remember* in this sense translates to God preparing to act on His promises. Even more important, God *remembering* confirms His covenant promises with His people. By giving Samuel to His people, He preserved and protected them. Samuel was to be the priest who would choose the kingly line that gave us Jesus (Ligonier Ministries, 2019).

True to His word, God helped Hannah conceive, and she bore a son. She named him Samuel, which means "I asked the Lord for him." And true to her word, Hannah gave Samuel back to the Lord for service. What a beautiful faithfulness she mirrors back to the Lord by saying, "You are worth ten sons. Now here's my only son."

The Shunammite Woman

The Shunammite woman was a wealthy woman. She and her husband owned a house large enough to provide hospitality for the prophet Elisha and his servant, Gehazi, during their visits to her town. She was eager to serve and care for them on their travels. She's another character whose birth name we are not told, perhaps because what was more memorable was her generosity.

Elisha took notice and wanted to repay her kindness. He offered to speak to the authorities on her behalf as a thank you gift. Kind of a strange way to thank someone, right? This suggestion implied that he thought she was in danger or needed his influence for protection. She was an infertile woman in ancient times, and commentaries suggest her husband was advanced in age. Should she be a widow with no heir, she would be quite vulnerable. The authorities could be useful by offering a decree to protect her home and land should she become widowed. She declined his offer with, "'I have a home among my own people'" (2 Kings 4:13 NIV). In my mind this would translate to, "I've got my own life. I'm fine. I'm wealthy. I don't need the help." I wonder if over time she had learned to build her life outside her desire to have children. I can relate to this, as there were seasons where I ceased putting my life on hold for the pursuit of a baby. I became frustrated with the fertility and adoption plans that seemed to eat up every minute, every bit of joy and hope. So I tried to build plan B distraction plans to allow myself other avenues of value, security, and hope. I numbly pushed through the steps of fertility treatment plans with low expectations. I learned to overprotect my heart. I applied for an MBA program, I over-engaged myself in work, and I took a leadership role in my Bible group. I wanted to show I was strong in other ways. I refused to stop my own self-constructed, very important, busy life for just a slim chance of a family. It was better to remain distracted, identified by other achievements, to avoid allowing myself to feel the weight of the grief and fear that having another baby might never happen.

Maybe the Shunammite was aware of her vulnerable state. Maybe she struggled to bring up this unspoken prayer. I understand everyone has their own level of openness when it comes to sharing their struggles. And the desire to be open or closed may change every day. Sometimes, the pain is so faith shattering and deep, it's best not to touch it, let alone allow someone else to look at it. When others look at it, it can feel as if they are using a magnifying glass. The last thing I needed was someone to look into that painful chasm, whatever their motivation, because it would completely derail the day in front of me.

Other times, we put up a shield or a mask. I couldn't risk disrupting someone else's life with my own. Too personal. Too painful. Too heavy to share. But often, I needed the help of a healing touch, word, or thought. *I'm fine,* I'd tell myself. *Really, it's fine.*

So Elisha scratched his head and asked, "What can be done for her?"

His servant replied, "She has no son" (2 Kings 4:14 NIV).

Wow, I've been there. Sometimes it felt so painstakingly obvious that I didn't have any children. My husband and I had been married for well over four years. I was *that* age. I was starting to be *past* that age. I was well-established in my career. We had purchased a home, moved closer to family. Maybe it was the way I gazed at families with young children. Maybe it was the way I teared up or became silent when plans for the next year were discussed at family parties. Would there be a chance for a baby next year, or would we give up? Would it ever be possible to have a baby in my arms?

It felt like everyone, those who knew my story and even those who didn't, were looking at me, pinning that label on me. The label read "Anticipate hard conversations." Broken, sad, lost, a liability, soul-draining, unreliable, unstable. I read it in their eyes when they asked for updates. I saw it from family members who appeared uncomfortable when I mentioned our babies in heaven. I felt it in the exclusions from gatherings that happened "last minute" when our invitation was "lost." But in painful hind-sight, it felt like I was avoided and identified by something I had little to no control over. *She has no son* … and my own addition, "she would give anything to have one."

Elisha told her, "'About this time next year you will hold a son in your arms.' 'No, my lord!' she objected. 'Please, man of God, do not mislead your servant!'" (2 Kings 4:16 NIV).

The Shunammite woman struggled to believe him, just like many of us would. But her unimaginable dream did come true: She had a son, and he grew to an age where he could be a little helper to his daddy. One day, while he was out in the fields with his father, he sustained an injury to his head, and he was brought to his mother's lap where he died. She laid him in Elisha's bed and immediately went in search of Elisha. She didn't even tell her husband. When he inquired why she was leaving the house, she gave no indication that their son's body lay lifeless in the house. She just saddled up and made the trip, which was estimated to be about twenty miles. When she approached Elisha, he knew by her appearance something was off. His servant Gehazi got to her first inquiring if something was wrong, and she said no.

She. Said. No. Everything was fine.

She hid it from Gehazi. This is the second time she hid her problems from someone.

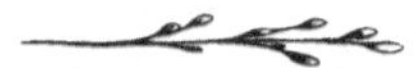

Grief makes us do funny things, doesn't it? There are times many of us feel like we can't share. But there are seasons when we need to be gently asked more than once if we are okay. Many of us tend to say, "I'm all right," when we're truly not. If you are the supportive friend or family member, you may be tempted to accept that response at face value or feel unsure about probing further because, who knows what kind of emotional reaction you might get? In *not* asking, you may feel like you are providing protection from triggering or from an emotional response. I had family members who were told not to ask me about our struggles to avoid discomfort—theirs or mine. Other loved ones had decided for me that it would be best to avoid the discussion altogether.

A friend of mine went through every cycle of IVF her body would allow until she had no embryos left. She and her husband decided this would be where the road ended for them. They were devastated and reeled with how to share this news. She decided to write her family members a letter with the details in hopes they could support and pray for them. This also freed her from having to repeat the painful story over and over to each group. When she shared her plan with her mother, her mother criticized her for oversharing information that was too personal. Deep grief spiraled to shame as she felt like her story needed to be hidden from those she longed to love her most.

Supporting a loved one walking through infertility is going to feel very uncomfortable. Your relationship is going to endure some pain points, if it hasn't already. Not forcing a conversation may feel protective, but the thing is these unending cycles of negative pregnancy tests, IVF cycles, loss of our babies, and not being chosen as a parent engulfs our lives. Every minute, that desire and those losses sit on the big screen in our mind on an unending loop. Talking about it doesn't bring grief to the front of mind: Trust me, it's already there. You will not help your loved one process their grief by pretending it doesn't exist. Because like the Shunammite woman, many of us survive our days by wearing a mask for those around us. To make it easier on you and, in many cases, on us, too. Be a safe place for your loved one to feel like they can take the mask off. It can be uncomfortable for some to talk about the things we go through. But you can sit with me. Tell me that you see me. Tell me you don't know what to say. Tell me you are praying. Tell me your heart is broken.

When the Shunammite woman reached Elisha, the grief dam broke. She was so distressed she couldn't speak. Somehow, Elisha knew something happened to the boy and sent speedy Gehazi ahead of him with his staff to heal the boy. Gehazi laid the staff on the dead boy, but it didn't work. Elisha later followed into the house to help. He went into the room, shut the door, and spread his own body over the child. Mouth to mouth, eyes to eyes, and hands to hands, and the child came to life.

Friends, this was an amazing miracle. We see that the power to bring someone to life could not be transferred through something that was not living, like a staff. It's not as though that staff didn't have the ability to do miracles. Previously, the staff had parted the waters of the Jordan not once, but twice (2 Kings 2:8, 14). However, the staff never brought a dead person to life. Life was only brought to the child by the warmth and stretching out of another human being.

Who is that for you? Who has brought warmth and life to you at a time that felt like death, even for just a moment? Perhaps it's a person who remembers your story when you feel forgotten. Or a person who offers intercessory prayer. What "staff" or other inorganic thing have you accepted for comfort in place of true healing? Is it the treatments you take? The mind-numbing, yet distracting television binges? Anything that we look to for comfort in these times that is not of the Lord represents that staff. It will not bring what is dead in you to life or bring peace to your situation. Rather, it delays the true healing process. Wait for the Healer, friend. The One who brings life and has already stretched Himself out for you on a cross.

Elizabeth

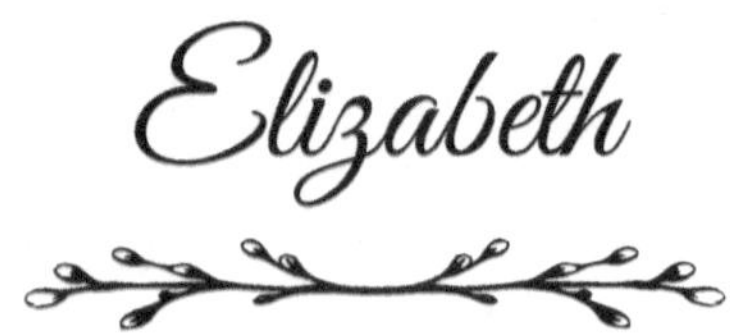

Luke 1:5-80

*E*lizabeth might very well be one of the most righteous, God-loving women that we will study. She was a genuine servant in the kingdom of God. In many ways, her story intimately overlaps Sarah's, as she did not conceive until she was well past fertile age. Elizabeth was thought to be somewhere around sixty years of age and described as "very old" (ouch) when she was introduced in the Bible. I think it's safe to assume she was post-menopausal and unable to get pregnant. We know from the Scriptures that the cause of her infertility was likely related to her own reproductive health. Baffling. A woman of God, infertile, a dedicated servant, shamed, the wife of a priest, stripped of the joy of motherhood.

Elizabeth and Zechariah, her husband, were both of priestly generations. Zechariah actively practiced as a priest and his heritage was of the division of Abijah. Abijah, as in the King of Israel, grandson of Solomon. The Bible tells us they were righteous in the sight of God, observant of His commands, and blameless.

Again, the Bible proves to us that infertility is not divine punishment, but that didn't excuse Elizabeth from social humiliation. Elizabeth was disgraced among her people (Luke 1:25). For her to identify as such and for the Bible to record it, I can only imagine the shame she endured over the years of her life. Disgraced. She had seen her season of fertility come and go. I think it was safe to say she was whispered about in the temple and in the community. Did her sisters in the temple divert their eyes when they saw her coming, not knowing what to say? Did they assume she had sinned? Did they wonder why God would not favor His servant? Was she afraid, as she had no heir to support her family?

Still, she and her husband dedicated their whole lives to serving the Lord. Their disappointment with God's plan did not keep them from His work. They trusted in His provision, His plan. Even if it meant heartbreak for them.

Luke 1 tells us Zechariah's division was on duty and he was the priest chosen to burn incense in the temple. This was a once in a lifetime opportunity. Lighting incense was an act of worship both for the priest and for the worshippers outside. The smell of incense signaled temple goers to communally pray and worship. It's likely as Zechariah lit the incense that filled that holy place, his own prayers also rose before the Lord. Most often priests would intercede for God's people and their salvation.

Is it possible that he was still praying for a son? Given his age, I think he likely had already come to peace with the fact he would not be a father. When no child came after years of prayer, he probably gave up. But God didn't. He heard every single prayer he had offered.

While Zechariah was in the holy place lighting the incense, an angel of the Lord appeared to him, standing just to the right of the altar scaring the daylights out of Zechariah. The angel told him not to be afraid and that his prayers had been heard. Elizabeth will bear a son.

I wonder if all this left Zechariah in a state of shock. His prayers had been clearly heard and responded to in angelic form. His past pleadings for a son and his current prayers for the salvation of God's people were answered all at once. His son—John the Baptist—would be the one to prepare the way for the Salvation of the World.

The angel identified himself as Gabriel and claimed his celestial authority as being in the direct presence of God. So, he was pretty much a VIP angel.

Gabriel instructed Zechariah to name this baby "John." John the Baptist, as we know him. Gabriel said, "He will be a joy and a delight to you, and many will rejoice because of his birth" (Luke 1:14 NIV). This part gets me every. Single. Time. Tears prick my eyes. This is it. This is the end of the road we all walk. This is where we all want to be. Zechariah didn't need to be told by some angel that his dream coming true would be a joy and a delight. He had waited so painfully long, that anticipation, that gift, would be inarguably the best thing that would ever happen to him. And it would be of no surprise that everyone around him would rejoice as well in the long-awaited, long-prayed-for gift of life.

Friends, I have a collection of pictures that I visit regularly of my two little guys just a few days in age and a few pounds in weight. In the photos, we are all gathered haphazardly in my bed. Maizey, the dog, sits behind them with an exhausted look on her face. The clock reads 3:22 a.m. They were up for their usual feed and I was fully enamored with them. I would sit and stare in disbelief at their little wrinkled old-man faces. No one would keep me from being mom paparazzi at any hour of the morning. They were and are my joy and my great delight. God saw fit that I would endure this journey for this very moment and many more to come.

Does that mean life was easy? That I no longer struggled with my identity, my story, postpartum anxiety, or any other troubles? No, absolutely not. But without a doubt, it changed my lens as a parent and my ability to trust God wholeheartedly.

How about for you or your loved one? Is there any chance that this long road produced a gift in you that you never would have experienced without this thorn? Would you have taken it for granted if it was just given to you? I can tell you this struggle has completely shaped our parenting. I am 100 percent confident that without this journey, I would have been selfish in my choices, less thoughtful in my parenting, less generous in my love, and further from God. It is only in humble gratefulness that I can see God sought to change my heart before He changed my family.

Gabriel went on to tell Zechariah that John would be great in the sight of the Lord, and the Holy Spirit would be in him before he was even born. John would be favored and would prepare the way for Jesus. It was all too good to believe it was real. So, Zechariah pointed out the obvious flaws in this plan. He said, "Wait a second. I'm old, and so is my wife. How's this going to happen?" Because he didn't believe Gabriel's words, Zechariah was no longer able to speak a word until the prophecy was fulfilled.

He left the temple and entered into the expectant crowd of worshippers. They understood something had happened because Zechariah had been in the temple a long time and now was silent, only able to motion with his hands. They assumed he had experienced some sort of vision. Later, he traveled home to be with Elizabeth and fill her in on the amazing news. But how did he tell her? Did he carefully write it in a long letter? Did he motion it out like charades? We don't know. But a miracle happened. Elizabeth became pregnant just as Gabriel said she would and went into seclusion for about five months.

I have exhaustively studied Zechariah and Elizabeth's life because I had many questions that the Bible doesn't fully answer. I wondered why God chose to take Zechariah's words as opposed to a different consequence. Being mute was a significant debilitation. In Zechariah's occupation, it would have been very hard to carry out priestly duties with no voice. Levitical priests served as intercessors for God's people. How can one intercede without spoken words? He probably struggled relationally due to the fact he couldn't engage in conversation. Of higher concern, how did he communicate with his wife? Did they have their own intimate sign language? Did he have a chalk board? Were they drawn together by quietude and reflection of what God had done? I wondered if perhaps in not speaking, he was forced to be a better listener, something his wife may have needed deeply. Maybe in his silence, he experienced a heightened perception of God's presence. He could see details others did not. Details we all take for granted, that are easily brushed over. Being mute may not have been the punishment it was thought to be, but rather a gift in disguise.

Interestingly, monastic silence is of the highest spiritual practice in religious tradition. What is its purpose? To grow closer to God. Zechariah's inability to speak prophetically mirrored the plight of God's people during that time. He couldn't speak, and they couldn't hear. The Israelites hadn't heard a word from the Lord for over 400 years. Many of them had grown far from God, impatient during this season of silence. They were pleading, begging for a king, a savior to rescue them from their political oppression. Zechariah served as an example of a new way of expectant waiting.

I wonder if God used the deafening silence to provide a platform for the crescendo of uninhibited worship to come. John's birth must have been an incredible celebration for Zechariah and Elizabeth. Everything they had hoped for their entire lives was born into miraculous existence in their advanced age. Zechariah would have wanted to shout from the rooftops what God had done. Yet God saw it fit to make him wait a little longer. How would he worship, and what would he say about this great gift that he waited for nine plus months to receive?

God could have taken away any of Zechariah's abilities. He could have taken away Zechariah's hearing, but then he wouldn't have been able to hear those first tiny shrieks when baby John entered the world. God could have taken his sight, but then Zechariah wouldn't have been blessed by the view of his wife's growing belly. God, in His goodness, chose to quiet Zechariah to allow him to marinate in awe and wonder. Allowing him space to reflect on how he would announce the greatest thing God had done in his life.

And what of Elizabeth? She went into a sort of isolation. I have several conclusions for why she decided to hide herself. I envision them both at home waiting together. Zechariah was lovingly faithful to her during all those years of infertility. He never left her. And Elizabeth never left him, even though he had doubted God's words through Gabriel. Was she embarrassed to be advanced in age and pregnant? Did she realize this was a high-risk pregnancy? Was this a self-directed bed rest she put herself on? She hid in seclusion for five months, which would equate to about twenty weeks into the pregnancy. Around that time, most pregnant women would be relatively out of the woods to miscarry. Is it possible Elizabeth had lost babies prior? Something had led her to wait it out with the Lord in private. I believe it was that she, too, struggled to believe. She needed God to show her day by day that He was good on His promises.

Looking over my years of infertility, I have been pregnant a total of six times with two successful pregnancies. I can tell you those times of being pregnant were tense, leaning on faith and the Lord. It was often difficult to be around others on a small-talk level when deep-level things were happening. I had a list of checkboxes running through my head. *Had I taken my meds, taken the scheduled vitamins, and timed the tests appropriately?* I internally assessed each physical symptom I was or wasn't having. People would ask me simple questions, and I would easily get confused, too absorbed by the daily checklist running a continuous loop in my head to answer. I struggled to be confident in my body because I had experienced so many losses. I would catch sight of my swollen belly in a sliding door, and the reflection downright flabbergasted me. My mind refused to register what my body was doing. I was anxious for women who announced their pregnancies early. This wasn't the life I knew.

I never chose to announce my pregnancies before the anatomy ultrasound, which usually occurred around twenty-weeks of pregnancy. My pregnancies were directed by weight-lifting limits, bed rest, progesterone shots, off-label intravenous infusions, and regularly scheduled monitoring. Having been pregnant so many times, my body showed signs early on. I would be sick as a dog and as tired as a granny, but still show up smiling in public like it was just another day. I pretty much lived in tunics and muumuus, hoping to remain unnoticed as babies filled and left my womb. I often held myself in seclusion and turned protectively inward, each day leaning on the Lord to continue to grow life in me.

I sought my small circle of friends who could be trusted with my messy emotions and endless checklists. I spent quiet intimate time with my husband, hoping and praying. I sought out God's Word and when I couldn't bring myself to read it, I had it read to me. In those times when I needed Jesus most, He provided the needed confidence that He would be faithful to be with me.

In our last stretch of the valley, we partnered with a reproductive clinic—CNY Fertility, over 600 miles away, known for its state-of the-art treatment and merciful out of pocket costs. We paid the cost to have our eggs carefully delivered across multiple state lines. Unfortunately, the timing coincided with the COVID-19 pandemic, complicating planning. My treatments were held with concerns of state lines being closed. Dr. Kiltz, a relentless advocate for infertile families, kept his clinic open when most had no choice but to close. We drove an extra two hours to the clinic because we could no longer cross the Canadian border. We spent multiple eerie nights alone in a local hotel to complete the necessary procedures to start IVF.

On Mother's Day, while snow flew over the highway, I carefully drove home from New York knowing I carried precious cargo. That IVF attempt resulted in another tragic chemical pregnancy. Our nerves were frayed knowing we only had a few precious eggs left, but we had made a decision to continue to the end. The phone call from the embryology lab came while I was playing ball with my sons.

"Mrs. LaVigne, we thawed your nine remaining eggs and none were viable, but one. We inseminated that one and you have only one embryo left to transfer."

I dropped to my knees. *One last chance.*

We decided for the sake of solidarity that our entire little family should go to New York for our last possible baby. The boys drew lots of maps and pictures of car trips to New York. My workload included care of COVID-19 patients, so while my husband navigated our car to New York from Michigan, I made calls to sick patients. We stayed in a cabin near Watkins Glen allowing us to explore Northern New York. Surrounded by the beauty of gorges and lakes, we soaked in the much-needed wonder for our Creator. My procedure was done in the usual skillful manner, but with a hurried undertone to avoid exposure to all in the room. I was alone for the procedure with exception of the doctor and nurse while my husband and boys played at a local park. We drove home together, holding hands with hearts laid open allowing God to lead in the road ahead.

In the days that followed, I hung on a thread between trusting God and spiraling down a path of doubt. One afternoon, while reading my Bible, a verse leapt from the page to my heart. "For he spoke and it came to be; he commanded, and it stood firm" (Psalm 33:9 NIV). I clung to it as we waited. The Lord whispered to my anxious heart, "You can trust Me to speak into your broken body. I will be sure it will stand firm. I have commanded it."

It was in those quiet whispers I learned to trust Him a little more. That He could handle the worries, the lists, the pain, the guilt. All the things I carried with me each day. He did not stand by wordlessly, waiting for me to do the right thing. I slowly realized that I had mischaracterized Him. I had placed Him in a box where I couldn't hear Him anymore. And in taking the sides off that box, each day I relied on Him a little more.

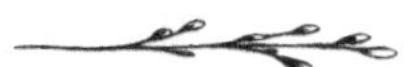

Elizabeth proclaimed, "The Lord has done this for me. In these days he has shown his favor and taken away my disgrace among the people" (Luke 1:25 NIV).

The Lord has done this for me.

I was driving through downtown Chicago in rush hour traffic trying to get to O'Hare for a flight to see a friend across the country. I was in blood work purgatory again, getting serial labs drawn. My blood work showed I was looking to be pregnant, but my HCG levels were not escalating in a gold standard way. At any point, a drop would indicate this would be another lost baby. I had to decide, should I take all of my meds with me on the plane (cooler, needles, etc.) or just assume the worst and leave it all at home? I hadn't gotten the call about my latest levels yet. I had to choose to trust that God knew what would happen, and that it was what was best for me. So, I schlepped all of my supplements, ice, cooler, syringes, and needles to the airport, all the while anxiously awaiting *the* call. In the middle of the Dan Ryan Highway in six lanes of traffic, the call came.

"Mrs. LaVigne, your beta-HCG has more than tripled. You are indeed pregnant. Let's schedule that ultrasound." *The Lord has done this for me.*

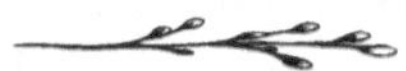

In the sixth month of Elizabeth's pregnancy, Gabriel appeared to Mary, telling her she was highly favored and that she would carry Jesus. He also shared the news that Elizabeth was pregnant. Elizabeth's pregnancy proved that no word from the Lord would fail. Mary could trust her own prophecy would be true. But she had to go and see for herself. So she hurried to Elizabeth and Zechariah's home, and when she greeted them, the baby did a happy dance in Elizabeth's belly.

Elizabeth was filled with the Holy Spirit and she was able to prophesy. Elizabeth said, "Blessed is she who has believed that the Lord would fulfill his promises in her!" (Luke 1:45 NIV). Elizabeth was encouraged, just as we should be, that the Lord was faithful in His promises to both of them.

This prompted Mary to prophesy through song about her soon-to-be son, Jesus. In her song, she recounted God's characteristics and names: Mindful, Mighty One, and Merciful. She remembered God's promise to Israel extending back to Abraham and his descendants. She was afraid but looked to the attributes of God to calm her anxious soul. It's in remembering His attributes that she reminded herself that He was in control. I encourage you to read Luke 1:46–53 when your soul needs anchoring and you need a reminder of who God is.

Mary stayed with Elizabeth for three months, likely until her due date. She was there for Elizabeth to lean on, confide in, and pray with. She probably did not stay for the birth, as this would make her unclean according to Jewish custom. Neighbors and relatives heard that the Lord had shown Elizabeth great mercy and they arrived to share in her joy, just as it was prophesied.

But poor Zechariah continued to be mute and his joy was

quieted even though the greatest answer to his prayers had arrived. When the baby was eight days old, it was time for his circumcision and naming ceremony. Relatives and friends suggested that Elizabeth name him after his father as was tradition for the first son. She insisted that he was to be named John prompting disagreement from friends and family. They went to Zechariah and tried to sign with their hands to express their concerns about this whole ordeal. Remember, the man could hear perfectly fine; he couldn't speak. (Insert head slap). Talk about being misunderstood. They didn't understand his limitations, or more likely were not around for the past several months, so they didn't know how to communicate with him.

I wonder why their relatives and neighbors were not aware of Zechariah's condition. It would seem that for the last half of Elizabeth's pregnancy they should have been aware. Wouldn't they have known how to communicate with him if they were relevant in their lives? Why were they not aware of his limitations? Did they just show up to see a miracle? It seemed family conflicts, struggles, and joy collided all at the same time.

My mind drifts back to varying seasons of support from my family. In the beginning, once it became clear we were having trouble conceiving, Brent and I met with them to share what we had been through. They quietly listened and agreed to pray. They said they didn't understand, but they would be there for us. And they were. The texts came, expressing support and lifting our souls. Greeting cards with Scriptures arrived in the mail. This was a healthier time for all of us. There was still a glimmer of hope. But no one knew this journey would stretch out for nearly a decade, becoming increasingly complicated and painful over the years.

During those ten years, my mom and dad divorced after forty years of marriage. The glue that held our family together had disintegrated. The protector of feelings and promoter of inclusion had left. The relationships I had grown up with became disoriented. Deep hurt and confusion seeped in as each of us learned how to be a broken family. We walked the uncharted territories of dysfunction, all learning how to protect our families as best as we knew how. Life kept life-ing, as it does, and the tension of lost dreams and waning family support wore on us. Eroding communication had made us less relevant in each other's stories. Our ears were wide open for words of support, but our family couldn't give the words our hearts needed to hear. Brent and I grew guarded, unsure of where we stood.

As fewer invites came for family gatherings, our fears grew that we were an emotional drain on an already depleted family. My dad waffled in the middle, just wanting everyone to get along. We tried several times to close the growing relational gap, but emotional capacity seemed to be at an all-time low due to this new grief. We felt like a liability on already strained connections. Excuses stood as walls where love would normally flow through. Hurt compounded on a perceived lack of support. So, when we went back to New York for our last embryo transfer, we kept to ourselves. Our hearts were too tender. All our energies, positive or otherwise, needed to be focused on necessary treatments and support for each other through another tenuous cycle. This was our last shot. We kept our circle small and for the first time it did not include our family members. We drew on other supports—close friends, church family, and accountability partners—to push us through. We spent time in the Word, and at the Lord's feet. I wonder if this time mirrored Elizabeth and Zechariah's solitude.

Do you harbor hurtful misunderstandings and strained relationships with those you need support from most? All while you keep on trudging through the dark night of the soul? Friend, this is by far one of the worst seasons I have been in. During this time of grief building on grief, we sought out high-quality therapy with a licensed counselor and relied heavily on the Lord to provide what we needed. We leaned into our small, precious circle of friends who loved us and loved Jesus. Day by day, our hope and faith grew. In our seclusion, we sought and found the Lord and flourished in His provided strength.

Over the next several months, forgiveness and healing sprang up. A sweet baby, Violet, would arrive, redeeming our faith and hope. My broken family, like Elizabeth's, gathered together in joy over a new miracle, seeing God's great mercy. Time and more time produced layers of healing and unspoken awareness that we all desperately needed.

If you are a supporter of someone on this journey, it's not for the faint of heart. Their story may not be one the Lord redeems quickly. Even more, redemption may not happen on this side of heaven. Expect to be uncomfortable. Expect brokenness and doubt to creep in. In their desire for preservation, your loved one may turn inward and isolate themselves from the protection of your relationship. Let them set the tone for what is needed from you and respect boundaries. Often, those struggling may need time to process their feelings, so talking things through may not be the solution. Of most importance, remain steadfast. Your presence and care remind them they are not alone on this journey.

For nine months, Zechariah held his long-awaited baby boy's name in his heart. He asked for a writing tablet and his tongue was set free the minute he wrote the words, "His name is John!" God gave him a second chance, and Zechariah was ready for it. He would shout it from the rooftops. He had waited three hundred days to be heard. He worshipped and then he prophesied.

How mind-blowing this must have been because there had not been public prophecy from any of God's people for 400 years. Now that John was born, the Holy Spirit that filled him was ignited all around him. Particularly in his father, who had burst forth in prophecy in song form (Luke 1:67–80). People from all over Judea heard about it, and hope spread. God's creation and people were desperate for a word from Him and Zechariah was desperate to praise God for what He had done. God used this moment to set the stage for Jesus, the ultimate fulfillment of prophecy.

Epilogue: Fractures Tell a Story

⁂

We had arrived in New York the day before. I had been resting all day after becoming sick from the injections used to prep my body. My head was foggy. I wasn't sure that I had the stamina to endure a hike, never mind any vigorous activity that didn't involve the four walls of a bathroom. We arrived at Watkins Glen State Park later than we hoped. After parking the car, I gingerly followed my husband and two rambunctious boys up the steps to the entrance of the park.

Upon entering, I realized that I was being ushered into a place of unexplainable beauty. Jagged rocks formed rugged side-walls and arches surrounding paths that led to small springs and waterfalls. The park is a 400-foot-deep gorge cut that was through rock by a stream formed by glaciers in the Seneca Valley. There are layers and layers of hard rock and soft shales showing the deep path the stream cut. I felt a hush of pure God-honoring worship, overwhelmed by the sight of His glory and perfect creativity.

We climbed the stairs and followed the rugged path laid out before us with several other tourists, taking pictures, putting our hands in the streams falling from rock formations towering high above us. We marveled at the stunning beauty of this place.

As we followed the path, I saw a sign that said, *"Fractures Tell a Story."* Beneath the heading it read:

> Notice the cracks, called joints, that run up the walls behind you. You can follow them through the creek bed and up the opposite wall. The joints represent a great continental collision that pushed up the Appalachian Mountains in Pennsylvania and the Allegheny Plateau…The tremendous pressure of the collision fractured the rocks of Watkins Glen and lifted the land skyward.
>
> (New York State Parks, Recreation, and Historic Preservation, 2020)

As I read this sign, I knew without doubt that the Lord was speaking directly to my heart, telling the story that was mine and would make sense later on. Knowing this was a holy moment, I took out my camera and snapped a shot to reflect on it later.

Friends, the last ten years of my life—the physical pain of endometriosis, the surgeries, surgical removal of my babies, IVF, adoption quests, and loss of my babies—has cut deep in a way that I, on my own, can never repair or comprehend. Just like that gorge, the fractures run deep and ragged. They show physical evidence of the intense pressure that my marriage, my home, my family, my life, and my faith endured. But the Lord in His immense goodness and His great authority saw fit that this would be my path. Pain carved a deep chasm that created a reliance on Him that could never be found on flat dry land. Faith showered from waterfalls of mercy and grace. The end result: a beautiful, fractured story lifted my life skyward in holy worship of Him.

The Lord, in His great wisdom, knew that our relationship would be redeemed under the pressure of great pain and sorrow. I had to choose to believe that He was at work in my circumstances to bring about redemption. His goal was always redemption. Those babies we lost, He holds them in heaven. My broken body will be redeemed upon the ushering in of the new heaven and new earth at Christ's return. When I chose to be obedient and trust the Lord, my relationship with Him, my husband, and others fell in line with His plan. My heart, again, was aligned with His and pointed the glory heavenward. This, friends, was the greatest miracle.

But even more, He knew that the physical evidence of His mercy—my sons and my soon-to-be daughter—would be visible for me for the rest of my life, and I would never be able to forget what He did for me. My Ebenezers.

So, I stacked stones there along with many others, knowing this was a turning point in my story. I promised I would never forget how my heart had changed.

Here's what I can't tell you: that your fractures, your deep grief, your increasing pressure will produce the same for you as they did for me. In fact, I can promise they won't, because while our paths may be the same, the outcome will be different. But there will be an end. There will be a sense of peace. Your heart indeed can be healed. And if you let Him lead you there, it will be the peace that passes understanding.

References

Bible Hub. "Wonderful." Expositor's Bible Commentary. Accessed January 14, 2026. https://biblehub.com/topical/w/wonderful.htm.

Eames, Christopher. "What Does the Name 'Sarai' Really Mean?" *Armstrong Institute of Biblical Archaeology*, December 21, 2022. https://armstronginstitute.org/818-what-does-the-name-sarai-really-mean.

Fleece, Esther. *No More Faking Fine: Ending the Pretending.* Grand Rapids, MI: Zondervan, 2017.

"God Remembers Hannah." Ligonier Ministries, March 29, 2019. https://learn.ligonier.org/devotionals/god-remembers-hannah.

Guzik, David. "Ruth 1 - Ruth's Journey." Enduring Word. https://enduringword.com/bible-commentary/ruth-1/.

Hayes, Cheree and Bible Project Team. "If God Remembers, Does He Also Forget?" *The Bible Project*, April 25, 2022. https://bibleproject.com/articles/if-god-remembers-does-he-also-forget/.

Mackie, Tim. Adam to Noah. Bible Project Classroom, 2024. https://bibleproject.com/classroom/adam-to-noah

New York State Parks, Recreation, and Preservation. "Fractures Tell A Story" sign. Glen Watkins State Park, Glen Watkins, NY. Viewed August 12, 2020.

Ortlund, Ray. *Good News at Rock Bottom: Finding God When the Pain Goes Deep and Hope Seems Lost.* Crossway, 2025.

"Our Mission." Resolve: The National Infertility Association, 2026. https://resolve.org/about-us/mission/.

Vroegop, Mark. *Dark Clouds, Deep Mercy: Discovering the Grace of Lament.* Crossway, 2019.

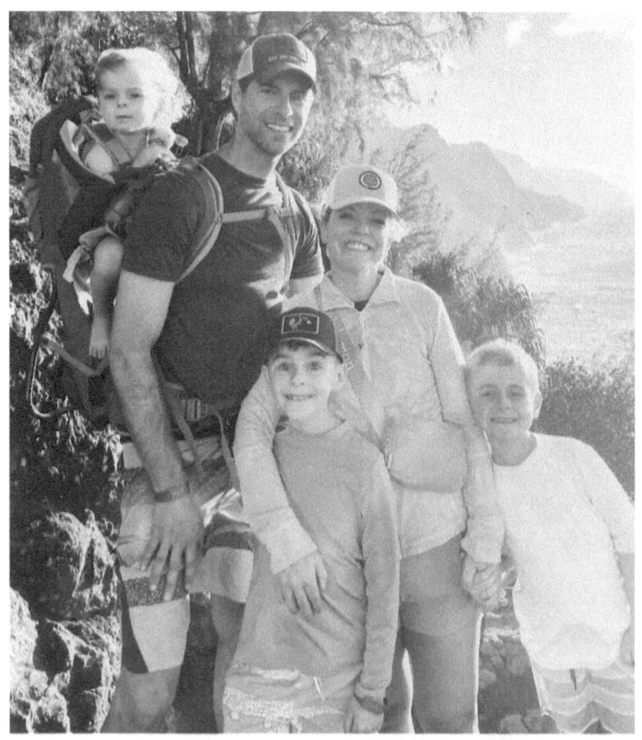

About the Author

Heather LaVigne is a Christ follower, wife, and mother through a little bit of science and a whole lot of Jesus. Heather was a Nurse Practitioner for 15 years before becoming an author, teacher, and ministry partner. With a deep love for scripture, it is her honor to walk alongside women in any stage of life, particularly those involving grief and loss. She is an advocate for those suffering through infertility, pregnancy, and child loss. She lives in Michigan with her husband, three children, two cats and rambunctious Labrador.

www.ingramcontent.com/pod-product-compliance
Lightning Source LLC
Chambersburg PA
CBHW021333060726
47591CB00006B/1996